The Healing Power of Touch – Guidelines for Nurses and Practitioners

Georg Seifert · Alfred Längler
Editors

The Healing Power of Touch – Guidelines for Nurses and Practitioners

External Applications in Pediatrics

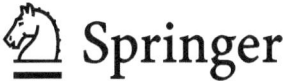 Springer

Editors
Georg Seifert
Department of Pediatrics
Division of Oncology and Hematology
Charité - Universitätsmedizin Berlin
Berlin, Germany

Alfred Längler
Department of Integrative Pediatric and
Adolescent Medicine
Gemeinschaftskrankenhaus Herdecke
University of Witten
Herdecke, Nordrhein-Westfalen, Germany

ISBN 978-3-030-85506-2   ISBN 978-3-030-85507-9   (eBook)
https://doi.org/10.1007/978-3-030-85507-9

This Springer imprint is published by the registered company Springer Nature Switzerland AG
The registered company address is: Gewerbestrasse 11, 6330 Cham, Switzerland

This book is dedicated to the work of nursing staff. Using touch on a daily basis, their tradition, expertise, and knowledge are passed hand-to-hand with tactile methods. We hope we have done this work justice. The ritual of embrocations and attention to the needs and bodies of the infirm affords the necessary space for health, well-being, and care: giving room for healing beyond what normal clinic treatment is able to provide.

Foreword

For humans, who belong to the family of nesting mammals, direct physical, bodily contact with other living beings of the same species is essential in every phase of life. Particularly during the early stages of human maturation, the body organism utilizes the biochemical signals derived from adequate physical contact for growth, relaxation, and healing. Benevolent and sufficient physical human contact is at no time more important than in early childhood. From a biological and psychological perspective, close human contact during this period has the same status as food. It is not only a guarantor for a thriving psychological and physical human development in the earliest phases of life but also facilitates essential processes of social bonding. Finally, adequate touch stimuli promote healing effects in every human being, the biochemical parameters of which we have yet to fully understand. For over a hundred years, we have known that the complexity and effects of interpersonal touch are far more important than just superfluous actions. Since the studies of H. Harlows or the reports of R. Spitz, it is known that humans, as nesting mammals, are essentially dependent on physical contact with other living beings of their kind. It has also long been known that touch stimuli can contribute to healing and recovery in people of all ages. One point has remained constant despite an ever-changing zeitgeist on touch; findings on healing touch stimuli were either ignored or even defamed in favor of technological and pharmacological hopes within medicine. However, in the last 30 years, the phenomenon of interpersonal touch in the medical context has experienced renewed attention and specialized scientific consideration. This is reflected in a growing number of basic scientific findings, but also concrete and clinically relevant findings replicated the world over. Whereas studies on the functioning of the human tactile system and on the effects of social touch stimuli were rather sporadic 30 years ago, publications on this topic fill entire rows of shelves or digital folders today. The increase in knowledge has thus reached a scope to which the extraction of the foundational essence in the form of specialized books is urgently necessary. Against this background, the authors of this book have attempted to summarize founded basic scientific facts, relevant subject-specific information, and, above all, practical aspects of body-oriented applications in the treatment of sick children and adolescents. With this book, the authors aim to close a publishing gap between the enormous number of scientifically based findings and knowledge of practical application. The streamlined and clear presentation of individual chapters are aimed directly at clinical users and also at parents caring for a sick child. With their texts, the authors not only convey knowledge from the practical spheres of healing professionals to medical laypersons but also assert confidence in the potentially healing effects of adequate and appropriate body stimulation. With their contributions, the authors raise awareness of the clinical possibilities for both children and adolescents, which can often be achieved through few means and with little time requirement. This book thus strengthens the perspective that therapeutically intended body interactions do not present a contradiction to other medical care, but can be a base and harmless part of the medical care of children and adolescents. I wish this book wide readership, attention, and scientific resonance so that not only practical-clinical practice is positively influenced, but also scientific curiosity about the mechanisms of therapeutic touch effects is fostered.

Martin Grunwald
Haptic Research Laboratory, University of Leipzig, Medizinische Fakultät
Paul-Flechsig-Institute for Brain Research
Leipzig, Germany
Martin.Grunwald@medizin.uni-leipzig.de

Preface

The idea to publish a book on external applications for children arose from a project in which we integrated selected naturopathic external applications from complementary medicine in a pediatric clinic for oncology and hematology at the Charité-Universitätsklinikum Berlin. This project showed that simple external applications can be very beneficial when used to complement/supplement conventional therapies, creating an integrative medicine in practice. We very quickly saw the beneficial effects. The results of our project reflected the experiences of many others as external applications have been used for centuries on children and adults.

What we refer to as "external applications" are therapeutic interventions that apply natural substances to the patient's body, often involving person-to-person skin contact. The effects of these applications unfold through attentive interpersonal touch as well as natural (mostly herbal) substance and temperature influences on the skin. The rhythmic application, the duration, and the post-treatment rest period also play an important role in the beneficial use of external applications.

In the case of children, external applications have a long tradition and are popular worldwide as home remedies, and their effects have been known since time immemorial. They are generally considered a safe alternative or supplement to many medications. Many of the readers will know of external applications from their own childhood. They are part of naturopathic oriented clinics and institutions and are also often used in private and home care.

The book is especially intended to provide nurses with supplemental therapeutic options for their daily care practice and to strengthen the competencies of parents who are caring for ill children.

Berlin, Germany   Georg Seifert
Herdecke, Nordrhein-Westfalen, Germany   Alfred Längler

Acknowledgments

We would like to thank Claudia vom Hoff-Heise for her incredible organizing talent in bringing all people and parts of this book together and without whom this project would not have been possible. For their linguistic expertise, we thank Sarah B. Blakeslee and Leanna Eaton for their English translation and editing of this book. A special note of thanks to the nursing staff at the Gemeinschaftskrankenhaus Herdecke for bringing their extensive and hands-on experience to light and on the page.

About this Book

The book is intended for healthcare professionals, therapists, and family caregivers interested in supplementing conventional pediatric care with external applications. It provides important background information meant to support the reader in understanding and contextualizing the potential benefits of integrating external applications into their care practice. The authors describe how children of different developmental stages can benefit from external applications such as rhythmic embrocations, baths, and compresses. The book is especially useful to caregivers because concrete instructions for implementing applications (including illustrations) are provided, specific external applications are recommended according to indication, and effects of substances (such as medicinal plants, oils, etc...) are explored.

A Note About Safety and Dosage

Medicine, like any science, is continually developing as research and clinical experiences expand our knowledge base. There has been relatively little scientific research into the treatment of children using natural substances. Knowledge in this area is largely based on the many years of clinical application experience by experts in the field. As far as this book mentions a dosage, a temperature, a duration of application, or age suitability, you as a reader can trust that the authors, the editor, and the publisher have taken great care to ensure the correctness and safety of the information. Care has been taken to ensure that all information is in accordance with the state of knowledge at the time of completion of the work, but the publisher cannot accept any responsibility for information on dosage instructions and forms of application. Each reader and user is urged to determine whether substances are suitable for use or whether there are contraindications by carefully examining the product information and package inserts of the substances and preparations used and, if necessary, after consulting a specialist. An examination of suitability and safety is particularly important when substances are used for the first time or if they are used rarely. Any application and dosage is at the users own risk. The authors and publisher appeal to each reader to notify the publisher of any inaccuracies or references.

The Structure of the Book

The first four chapters of this book present important background information meant to support the reader in understanding and contextualizing the potential benefits of integrating external applications into their care practice. Whereas Chaps. 5–7 provide more practical, hands-on information, including concrete instructions for implementation, application recommendations based on indications, and an exploration of substances used in external applications.

Chapter 2 provides a conceptual framework for understanding the historical origins of external applications anchored within traditional and complementary medicine, including a definition of health and health promotion according to salutogenetic principles. This chapter provides insights into the broad spectrum of effective factors of external applications used in pediatric care with a special emphasis on interpersonal attention and touch for promoting health, along with the chemical and physical effective factors of the applications themselves.

As almost all of the applications included in this book involve touching a patient's skin, it is essential to fully understand how the skin develops, its structure, and its functions in the human organism. Chapter 3 helps the reader to come to a deeper anatomical and functional understanding of skin. It goes further to elaborate how the peculiarities of children's skin and their stages of development have direct implications for the implementations of external applications.

Chapter 4 is devoted to exploring a phenomenological perspective of the body, moving away from the categorization of the body as an object by introducing readers to the concept of the lived body. The author shows the reader that the therapeutic effects of external applications can only be truly evaluated when the schema begins with the acknowledgment of each individual body as a subject, through which the world is perceived.

Readers will find detailed guidance on application techniques in Chap. 5. This chapter provides concrete instructions for the implementation of external applications, including descriptions, lists of materials needed, and illustrations to help the reader understand and apply each technique.

Chapter 6, Indications is the heart of the book. Indications from a wide spectrum of pediatric care, including pediatric surgery, psychiatry, oncology, intensive care, neonatology, and around child development, are sorted by indication groups. Many typical indications are listed and recommendations for applications, contraindications, age suitability, dosages, and, where applicable, temperature of applications are provided.

External applications generally use teas, oils, essential oils, minerals, and/or other animal substances. The final chapter of this book helps the reader understand more precisely which substances can be used for which indication. Each substance is presented through a fact sheet which includes the classification, origin, composition, a brief overview of its tradition as a remedy, effects, range of use, external forms of application, and contraindications. Finally, various finished preparations and their supply sources are mentioned.

When all chapters are taken together, this book presents the reader with both a comprehensive introduction to the theoretical background and naturopathic origins of external applications while also providing the practical and concrete information necessary to integrate external applications into their daily care practice.

Contents

1

Georg Seifert and Alfred Längler

Why is touch so important? The sense of touch is the first sense which develops in the unborn child. At as early as 6–8 weeks gestation, an unborn child experiences touch in the womb and even after birth, touch continues to have a tremendous impact on their long-term health and psyche. We need the touch of our parents and our closest relatives to stay healthy. Children receive loving touch from parents, grandparents, and family for granted. The older we get, the less touch happens naturally and even hugs have become increasingly rare in a digitalized world. Yet touch is as important as the air we breathe. A lack of touch not only leads to stress, high blood pressure, or immune deficiency but can also lead to life-threatening conditions, as shown in animal experiments. From many studies with orphaned children, we know how dramatic the effects of a lack of physical and emotional attention can be. The younger the children, the greater the negative repercussions from experiencing a lack of touch. Conversely, this means that the positive effect of touch can also be of great therapeutic importance.

The aim of this book is to open up the therapeutic potential of touch and to present a wide range of external applications suitable for children and youth. From our clinical perspective, the effects of the therapeutic possibilities described in this book are particularly impressive with children who are ill. The authors of this book offer a wide variety of applications, ranging from the most simple—lasting only a few minutes, which can be implemented by laypersons (especially parents) after brief

G. Seifert (✉)
Integrative Medicine in Pediatric Oncology, Department of Pediatric Oncology and Hematology, Charité – Universitätsmedizin Berlin, Berlin, Germany
e-mail: Georg.seifert@charite.de

A. Längler
Department of Pediatric and Adolescent Medicine, Gemeinschaftskrankenhaus Herdecke, Herdecke, Germany
e-mail: a.laengler@gemeinschaftskrankenhaus.de

1

instruction, to more elaborate complex rhythmic embrocations that require specific training and expertise.

Experiences in family medicine clearly show how effective even simple external applications can be and point to the importance of touch. Take, for example, the relatively common, complex initial conversation with parents who have received a momentous diagnosis for their child. It is not uncommon for the simple act of placing a hand on their shoulder to provide more peace and security than the actual two-hour educational talk itself. Other examples can be found in pediatric oncology where, in addition to questions about effectiveness of various techniques and substances, the subjective experience of the patient (and practitioner) also plays an important role in the indication and successful implementation of external applications. In day to day clinical practice, it is a regular occurrence for patients to indicate acutely and subjectively an improvement of their symptoms after experiencing external applications. Such was the case for a 14-year-old patient with neutropenic pneumonia after chemotherapy for an Ewing's sarcoma. Despite antibiotic and inhalation therapy, the patient had persistent tachydyspnea (with adequate peripheral oxygen saturation) and intermittent episodes of coughing. It was striking for us to experience the subjectively positive effect of applying a wrapped ginger flour compress to his chest. After performing the chest wrap daily, he regularly reported feeling that he could breathe better and seemed less strained. For several hours afterwards, he had fewer coughing attacks and was able to relax significantly. His breathing frequency usually became calmer. This is not proof of efficacy in an objective sense, but it does show how these and similar nursing applications can be experienced as helpful and relieving by an individual patient in a specific situation. The subjective experiences of patients are a central point that is becoming increasingly important in medical science, in the sense of patient centricity.

We hope that reading this book will provide you with ideas and suggestions to make your everyday therapeutic work more varied and enrich your diagnostic repertoire to the benefit of the young patients you care for. We also see the potential for the information included to help strengthen the competences of parents caring for ill children.

Conceptual Framework and Effective Factors of External Applications

2

Inga Mühlenpfordt and Georg Seifert

2.1 Introduction

Interpersonal affection and touch play an essential role in everyday human social interactions from birth. Although their healing capacities are obvious, they have been given surprisingly little importance in pediatric practice in Western countries in recent decades. External applications use natural substances; the effects of temperature; and touch techniques to create a special way of caring for and interacting with patients. Evidence-based medical therapies and nursing techniques can thus be usefully supplemented to provide comprehensive support for the individual healing process in children.

2.2 External Applications: Anchored in Traditional Medicine

Modern external applications are inspired by experiential knowledge from various currents of traditional medicine. For thousands of years, they have been part of the repertoire of common remedies in the form of embrocations, massages, wraps, washes, and baths. The first references to the use of compresses can be found around

I. Mühlenpfordt (✉) · G. Seifert
Department of Pediatric Oncology and Hematology, Charité – Universitätsmedizin Berlin, Berlin, Germany
e-mail: Inga.muehlenpfordt@charite.de; Georg.seifert@charite.de

G. Seifert, A. Längler (eds.), *The Healing Power of Touch – Guidelines for Nurses and Practitioners*, https://doi.org/10.1007/978-3-030-85507-9_2

1500 years B.C. in Egypt, where heated Nile mud was used as a healing poultice. *Hippocrates* (460–380 BC) described medicine as "the art of touch" handed down from the doctor and teacher. In *Kneipp Therapy* (after the naturopath Sebastian Kneipp, 1821–1897), compress applications occur as a component of hydrotherapy [1]. The founders of *Anthroposophic Medicine*, the spiritual scientist Rudolf Steiner and the physician Ita Wegmann, integrated external applications at the beginning of the twentieth century as a component in their range of methods based on natural science-oriented medicine [2]. Today, external applications are predominantly found in private, domestic use. In complementary systems of naturopathic medicine as well as in integrative medicine, external applications based on experiential knowledge continue to be in use today.

Applications are often performed by trained nurses or other trained caregivers. Particularly when treating children, they offer the opportunity to reduce anxiety and increase wellbeing during other medical treatments. In unsettling situations and unfamiliar clinical environments, they can provide respite. There is evidence that pediatric patients enjoy external applications and find them supportive. In stressful situations, external applications are also particularly valued by parents and found to be calming, relaxing, and pain relieving for their child [3]. After appropriate training, parents and other caregivers can be involved in the applications or perform them themselves.

2.3   Conceptual Framework of External Applications

External applications can be used in addition to other medical and nursing methods. According to their medical-historical origins, external applications are based on a so-called *holistic understanding of health*. According to this, the human being is not only considered to have a physical level but also a soul and spirit. Each of these parts influences the others; and all parts can be addressed together in medical treatments that promote health and healing [2]. External applications can be aimed at specific symptoms, while also *promoting health* and stimulating healing processes. At the same time, the details of execution can be tailored to the *individual needs of* the patient and their *social environment* (see Fig. 2.1).

2.3.1   Holistic Understanding of Health

Whereas science-based medicine often places great emphasis on the established diagnosis and its specific treatment, the theoretical framework and assumptions about the goals of treatment in traditional and complementary medicine often place

Fig. 2.1 Framework of external applications

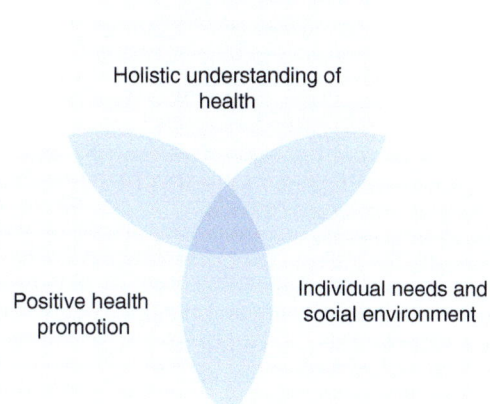

Holistic understanding of
health

Positive health
promotion

Individual needs and
social environment

attention on the whole person. Medical success is achieved not only with the disappearance of specific symptoms, but also through holistic personal development [4, 5]. According to the approach of holistic medicine, the whole person is considered and treated in the context of his or her life.

A recurring idea in the history of medicine is that equilibrium or balance constitutes health. Different parts and functions of the human body and mind thus intertwine and harmonize with each other. The idea of balance is strongly represented in several non-Western medical traditions. In Western medicine, the idea of balance was systematically developed in the Hippocratic and the Galenic schools (Hippocrates 460–380 BC and Galen 129–216/7 AD). The concept of equilibrium is also used in modern Western thought—especially in physiology. For example, Walter Cannon (1871–1945), in his work on homeostasis (1932), described in detail how the various physiological functions of the body control each other and interact in feedback loops to prevent major disturbances [6]. According to this holistic view, health is the result of successful self-regulating internal activity and the constant (re)establishment of harmony between the functions of body. Illness can be understood as the expression of a system imbalance. The goal in holistic medicine is to restore balance by stimulating different processes in the body. The entire constitution of patients is strengthened by taking into account the emotional, physical, social, mental, and spiritual dimensions [7].

2.3.2 Positive Promotion of Health: Focus on Salutogenesis and Consideration of the Context

To support health, it is worthwhile not to focus exclusively on a patient's existing pathology or symptoms of disease. Rather, there is an opportunity to view the human being as a complex system, taking into account health-promoting and preventive as well as curative and rehabilitative ideas and practices [8]. In this sense, *salutogenetically* oriented treatments focus on positive health promotion. The therapeutic goals of health-promoting applications are to recognize and stimulate self-efficacy and self-regeneration by enabling autonomous self-regulation [9] as well as psycho-emotional and spiritual self-regulation. This also means that medical treatment should strengthen a *sense of coherence by* motivating patients and the environment to cope with the disease situation (meaningfulness), enabling understanding the disease and accompanying factors (comprehensibility), and providing resources for coping with the applications (manageability) [8].

The context of the medical treatment [10] as well as the meaning attributed to the application [4] may have an influence on the effect of treatments themselves. These nonspecific influences are usually referred to as *placebo effects in* medical research and practice. They operate in all age-groups via the same mechanisms, the effectiveness of treatments can be enhanced by: the presence of realistic expectations of an effect; practitioners who invest time in the relationship with the patient; and respond to individual needs and the presence of conditioning mechanisms. Children and adolescents also show high response rates to placebo effects [11].

Despite the establishment of evidence-based practice, elements of health care today can still allow for cultural practice and rituals. Through the use of certain touch and movement techniques, substances, and temperatures, as well as the post treatment rest periods associated with the applications, external applications harbor certain treatment procedures that can make them a ritual. Health care practice can be complemented by effective rituals that have a reinforcing placebo effects [10, 12].

External applications exhibit a wide range of nonspecific effects, which depend upon the patient-practitioner relationship and the patient's belief in their effectiveness. The overall effectiveness of external applications is increased through the establishment of rituals, interpersonal attention and sympathy, detailed diagnostic measures, and explicit reflection on the complaints related to the applications. In addition, when the external applications are based upon and are tailored to the patient's complaints, it can change the patient's view of their own illness and symptomatology as well as of their fears and expectations.

2.3.3 Individual Needs and Social Environment

In the medical care and treatment of children, the simultaneous collection of information in two areas is required. One is the *disease itself,* which includes symptoms, indicators, examinations, and clinical management. The other is the *subjective view on the disease*, that is, the patient's concerns, expectations, feelings, and thoughts. It is not only the somatic indicators of health that are important, but also the subjective health and health-related quality of life of the patient. The patient's social environment also determines the way the patient is treated: treatment providers, parents, and other people involved in the care-giving influence the handling of diseases. How a patient gets along with other people and copes with everyday life is also relevant [13–15].

Illness and symptoms of illness often place pediatric patients and their parents and caregivers in stressful situations, triggering stress and negative emotions. Research in recent years points to the importance of strengthening personal family and other social resources to manage children's health risks and impairments. By means of medical-therapeutic treatments, patients and those surrounding them can be empowered to do things for themselves, bringing some sense of relief. In terms of family-centered care, the family environment of pediatric patients is considered an important constant, whose inclusion in the care processes, especially in children, leads to the patient receiving a higher quality of care, better accepting of applications and gaining confidence in the effectiveness of treatments [16].

In addition to the well-being of the patient, the well-being of the parents and other caregivers also plays a central role in the healing process. The familiy members often have to take care of the child full-time during the time of therapy, in the clinic setting or at home. If the child's illness is prolonged, emotional uncertainty, pressure, and despair characterize daily life, and helplessness and hope can rise and fall. In this situation, moments of hope, relaxation, and stress relief are very valuable for the parents and care-givers as well. A first impulse in response to stress is often seeking attention and a desire to be cared for, but there is also an impulse on the opposite side to care for those in need of help (*Tend and Befriend Model*) [17]. Parents and caregivers of pediatric patients may feel a desire to contribute in helping to manage a condition and symptoms of illness [3]. To address these impulses, family members can be involved in implementing external applications. After appropriate training, it is also possible for the applications to be used outside of a clinical setting, e.g. at home.

External applications provide an opportunity to address both the illness and symptoms as well as the context of the illness in a patient-centered manner. They provide a framework for incorporating individual patient needs and preferences into the selection of applications and for fine-tuning applications to meet the needs of the child patient. As parents and caregivers can also be involved in the implementation of external applications, they can also contribute to activating a patient's social resources.

2.4   Effective Factors of External Applications

External applications combine interpersonal attention and touch, pressure and rhythmic movements with temperature, and fragrance effects of substances on the skin, through the use of tempered water, essential oils, and natural substances. External

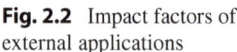

Fig. 2.2 Impact factors of external applications

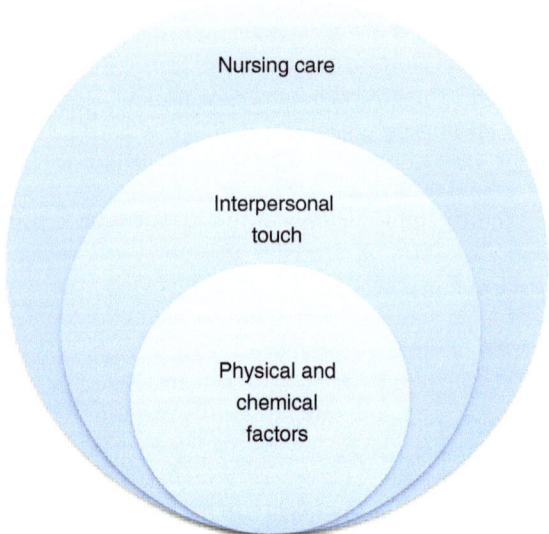

applications are thus characterized by a spectrum of effective factors that can vary and contribute to the effect of the applications. Influencing the effect of external applications are, on the one hand, the social factors of *nursing care* and social support as well as interpersonal *touch*. Haptic-tactile stimuli on the skin have an effect through the use of certain movement sequences and the locality of the application. Temperature works as a *physical stimulus* and substances work through their *chemical influences* and develop their effect during external applications (see Fig. 2.2).

The choice of application depends on the indication and any diagnosis that may be present. The physical as well as the psychological condition of the patient provide additional indications as to which application is appropriate. The individual constitution, as well as one's own wishes and goals with regard to a therapeutic intervention, should be considered in advance of any application. In the case of medical care treatment and support of children, applications should also be coordinated with the parents and other caregivers.

2.4.1 The Potentials of Social Proximity in Nursing Care

Modern western medicine offers numerous successful treatment options in pediatrics. At the same time, modern western medicine is often criticized for having lost much of its human touch. Treatment concepts are perceived as increasingly impersonal [14]. Attention and social closeness can help reduce the risk of developing physical and mental illness and promote health and longevity. Interpersonal affection is therefore considered important for promoting health, for example, to regulate emotions in the social environment and thus conserve somatic and neural resources (*Social Baseline Theory*) [18].

A child who is treated by external applications is in close contact with the person performing the treatment. During the applications, children often experience special attention and loving care. Established medical and nursing practices can be supplemented by the valuable actions and social aspects of external applications as an important part of general pediatric patient care in the clinical setting. The applications create space for attention to be paid to the patient's concerns and worries in the context of physical experiences. At the same time, external applications hold the potential to increase patient trust in those administering the treatments and foster the patient-caregiver relationship. In this way, young patients can experience support, gather strength and energy.

2.4.2   Health Promotion Via Interpersonal Touch

The sense of touch is the first of the senses to develop in the human body before birth. Experienced through a complex system of nerve fibers on the skin, the sense of touch is of great importance to perception and social interaction [19]. Touching the skin with a certain rhythm and pressure stimulates pressure receptors, which can lead to positive affective valence by stimulating C-tactile fibers in the skin, in particular via haptic-tactile perception. This may lead to activation of the vagus nerve, through which the positive effects of touch may be mediated [20, 21]. At the hormonal level, touch may inhibit the release of cortisol, whereas touch may promote the release of dopamine, serotonin, and oxytocin. Oxytocin, in particular, has been associated with modulating pain, increasing wound healing, and reducing stress [22–25]. In summary, touch can thus have healing effects on the body.

The potential of touch interventions is well known in research. Interpersonal touch is associated with healthy development and with promoting health and immune function in general. Positive psychological effects of touch are evident in improved emotion regulation, increased attention, and reduced levels of stress, depression, and anxiety [20, 26]. The literature also suggests that massage therapies have positive effects on various childhood conditions [27]. Touch can create and strengthen the emotional regulatory capacity of the receiving patient. This reduces the need to invest one's own regulatory resources, which can reduce anxiety in particular [18]. Touch can therefore be of great importance in situations where individuals need social support and protection.

Touch-based external applications offer an opportunity to enter into targeted interpersonal contact via touch. Particularly in embrocations and massages, special importance is attached to the movement sequences as well as the rhythm and the speed of execution. Likewise, the intensity of pressure and duration of treatment and appropriate post-treatment rest periods are considered carefully. In some applications, specific rhythms are used to stimulate nerve fibers and regulate the bodily functions, such as metabolism, blood circulation, peristalsis, and respiration [28].

2.4.3   Physical and Chemical Factors: Use of Active Substances and Temperature

An important part of the effect of external applications results from the specific substances used and the temperature at which they are applied. In external applications, natural substances are used, including essential oils obtained from plants. These substances can be used in different forms and dosages; their recommended use is usually based on many years of practical experience. What they have in common is the aromatic effect on the skin, and through the scent of the essential oils themselves. The substance application temperature can match the patient's body temperature or be warmer or colder, depending on the desired effect [29]. In addition to the indication, the patient's own preferences and habituation are important and should be considered during the selection of substances and temperatures of application.

Essential oils can be absorbed by smell as well as through the skin. Studies in recent years have shown that olfactory and taste receptors are not exclusively found in the nasal olfactory epithelium or in taste bud cells. Receptors have rather been identified in a number of extra-nasal and extra-oral tissues involved in various biological processes. Research suggests that the receptors are involved in muscular regeneration, regulation of inflammatory processes, and energy metabolism, among others [30, 31]. Fragrances and temperature effects can also influence the release of endogenous opioids, for example, pleasant warmth and familiar odors can promote the release of oxytocin [25].

References

1. Sonn A (2004) Pflegepraxis: Wickel und Auflagen: Alternative Pflegemethoden erfolgreich anwenden [Wraps and compresses. Using alternative care methods successfully]. Thieme
2. Kienle GS, Albonico H-U, Baars E, Hamre HJ, Zimmermann P, Kiene H (2013) Anthroposophic medicine: an integrative medical system originating in Europe. Global Adv Health Med 2(6):20–31. https://doi.org/10.7453/gahmj.2012.087
3. Stritter W, Rutert B, Eidenschink C, Eggert A, Längler A, Holmberg C, Seifert G (2021) Perception of integrative care in paediatric oncology-perspectives of parents and patients. Complement Ther Med 56:102624. https://doi.org/10.1016/j.ctim.2020.102624
4. Brown CK (1998) The integration of healing and spirituality into health care. J Interprof Care 12(4):373–381. https://doi.org/10.3109/13561829809024944
5. Krenner L (2019) Integrative medicine - rediscovering wholeness. In: Frass M, Krenner L (eds) Integrative medicine. Elsevier, Philadelphia, pp 3–21. https://doi.org/10.1007/978-3-662-48879-9_1
6. Nordenfelt L (2017) On concepts of positive health. In: Schramme T, Edwards S (eds) Handbook of the philosophy of medicine. Springer, Dordrecht, pp 29–43. https://doi.org/10.1007/978-94-017-8688-1_2
7. Hawks S (2004) Spiritual wellness, holistic health, and the practice of health education. Am J Health Educ 35(1):11–18. https://doi.org/10.1080/19325037.2004.10603599
8. Antonovsky A (1996) The salutogenic model as a theory to guide health promotion. Health Promot Int 11(1):11–18. https://doi.org/10.1093/heapro/11.1.11

9. Heusser P (1999) Academic research in anthroposophic medicine. Example of hygiogenesis: natural and spiritual scientific approaches to the self-healing power of the human being. Peter Lang

10. Kaptchuk TJ (2002) The placebo effect in alternative medicine: can the performance of a healing ritual have clinical significance? Ann Intern Med 136(11):817–825. https://doi.org/10.7326/0003-4819-136-11-200206040-00011

11. Weimer K, Gulewitsch MD, Schlarb AA, Schwille-Kiuntke J, Klosterhalfen S, Enck P (2013) Placebo effects in children: a review. Pediatr Res 74(1):96–102. https://doi.org/10.1038/pr.2013.66

12. Catanzaro AM (2002) Beyond the misapprehension of nursing rituals. Nurs Forum 37(2):17–27. https://doi.org/10.1111/j.1744-6198.2002.tb01194.x

13. Bullinger M (2002) Assessing health related quality of life in medicine. An overview over concepts, methods and applications in international research. Restor Neurol Neurosci 20(3–4):93–101

14. Levin DL, Todres ID (2006) History of pediatric critical care. In: Fuhrman BP, Zimmerman JJ (eds) Pediatric *critical care*. Elsevier, Amsterdam. https://doi.org/10.1016/B978-0-323-01808-1.X5001-9

15. Sullivan M (2003) The new subjective medicine: taking the patient's point of view on health care and health. Soc Sci Med 56(7):1595–1604. https://doi.org/10.1016/S0277-9536(02)00159-4

16. Harrison TM (2010) Family-centered pediatric nursing care: state of the science. J Pediatr Nurs 25(5):335–343. https://doi.org/10.1016/j.pedn.2009.01.006

17. Taylor SE, Master SL (2010) Social responses to stress: the tend and befriend model. In: Contrada R, Baum A (eds) The handbook of stress science: biology, psychology, and health. Springer, New York, pp 101–109

18. Beckes L, Coan JA (2011) Social baseline theory: the role of social proximity in emotion and economy of action. Soc Personal Psychol Compass 5(12):976–988. https://doi.org/10.1111/j.1751-9004.2011.00400.x

19. Montagu A (1971) Touching: the human significance of the skin. Columbia University Press, New York

20. Field T (2010) Touch for socioemotional and physical Well-being: a review. Dev Rev 30(4):367–383. https://doi.org/10.1016/j.dr.2011.01.001

21. Pawling R, Cannon PR, McGlone FP, Walker SC (2017) C-tactile afferent stimulating touch carries a positive affective value. PLoS One 12(3):1–15. https://doi.org/10.1371/journal.pone.0173457

22. Detillion CE, Craft TKS, Glasper ER, Prendergast BJ, DeVries AC (2004) Social facilitation of wound healing. Psychoneuroendocrinology 29(8):1004–1011. https://doi.org/10.1016/j.psyneuen.2003.10.003

23. Eliava M, Melchior M, Knobloch-Bollmann HS, Wahis J, da Silva Gouveia M, Tang Y, Ciobanu AC, Triana del Rio R, Roth LC, Althammer F, Chavant V, Goumon Y, Gruber T, Petit-Demoulière N, Busnelli M, Chini B, Tan LL, Mitre M, Froemke RC et al (2016) A new population of parvocellular oxytocin neurons controlling magnocellular neuron activity and inflammatory pain processing. Neuron 89(6):1291–1304. https://doi.org/10.1016/j.neuron.2016.01.041

24. Field T, Hernandez-Reif M, Diego M, Schanberg S, Kuhn C (2005) Cortisol decreases and serotonin and dopamine increase following massage therapy. Int J Neurosci 115(10):1397–1413. https://doi.org/10.1080/00207450590956459

25. Uvnäs-Moberg K (1998) Oxytocin may mediate the benefits of positive social interaction and emotions. Psychoneuroendocrinology 23(8):819–835. https://doi.org/10.1016/S0306-4530(98)00056-0

26. Holt-Lunstad J, Birmingham WA, Light KC (2008) Influence of a "warm touch" support enhancement intervention among married couples on ambulatory blood pressure, oxytocin, alpha amylase, and cortisol. Psychosom Med 70(9):976–985. https://doi.org/10.1097/PSY.0b013e318187aef7

27. Field T (2019) Pediatric massage therapy research: a narrative review. Children 6(6):78. https://doi.org/10.3390/children6060078

28. Bertram M, Ostermann T, Matthiessen PE (2005) Exploring Wegman/Hauschka rhythmic rubs. A structural phenomenological investigation. Nursing 18(4):227–235. https://doi.org/10.1024/1012-5302.18.4.227

29. Gündling A, Gündling PW (2011) Aromatherapy in pediatrics. Erfahrungsheilkunde 60(03):158–164

30. Lee SJ, Depoortere I, Hatt H (2019) Therapeutic potential of ectopic olfactory and taste receptors. Nat Rev Drug Discov 18(2):116–138. https://doi.org/10.1038/s41573-018-0002-3

31. Wölfle U, Elsholz FA, Kersten A, Haarhaus B, Müller WE, Schempp CM (2015) Expression and functional activity of the bitter taste receptors TAS2R1 and TAS2R38 in human keratinocytes. Skin Pharmacol Physiol 28(3):137–146. https://doi.org/10.1159/000367631

Human Skin

3

Christoph Schempp

3.1 Introduction

This chapter describes the anatomy as well as the physiological functions and development of the skin as an organ, but also the psychological elements and sensory touch. The sense of touch begins to develop during the embryonic stages and continues to develop throughout childhood. Skin plays an essential role in the proper functioning of the entire body and thus also for child development. The peculiarities of children's skin, and their stages of development, have direct implications for the implementations of external applications.

The skin is our largest sensory organ, its size and weight are more comprehensive than any other organ of the human body. The skin not only demarcates the body internally (mucous membranes) and externally but also has multiple physiological and psychosocial functions.

The human skin performs important functions for the human metabolism and immune system. It also has direct access to external sensations like no other organ of the human body. Temperature changes, radiation, and substances can act directly on the skin from the outside. While at the same time, the skin forms an important protective barrier between the organism and harmful environmental influences. The

C. Schempp (✉)
Department of Dermatology and Venereology, University Medical Center Freiburg,
University of Freiburg, Freiburg, Germany
e-mail: christoph.schempp@uniklinik-freiburg.de

G. Seifert, A. Längler (eds.), *The Healing Power of Touch – Guidelines for Nurses and Practitioners*, https://doi.org/10.1007/978-3-030-85507-9_3

skin is crucial for communication with the animate and inanimate environment. Through it comes the sense of touch, in which, for example, touch can be transmitted and perceived from one person to another.

3.2   Anatomy and Function of the Skin

A detailed account of the anatomical and functional threefold organization of the skin can be found in Bolognia and Fritsch [1, 2]. In the following, the morphological structure of the skin and the functional classification of the skin-associated immune system are briefly discussed.

3.2.1   The Epidermis

The human epidermis consists of only a few cell layers (Fig. 3.1). The metabolic activity of the epidermis is tightly regulated and greatly reduced compared to other tissues. Only the epidermal stem cells in the basal layer are capable of proliferation. In the epidermis, one stem cell re-enters the resting phase after the first cell division, while the other does not proliferate further after approximately two cell divisions, but instead undergoes various stages of differentiation starting in the stratum granulosum, which then leads to cell death in the upper stratum granulosum with the dissolution of the nucleus and fusion of the cell contents into the environment [2]. Thus, the upper third of the epidermis undergoes a continuous process of death (apoptosis). The dead keratinocytes, previously tightly bound together by

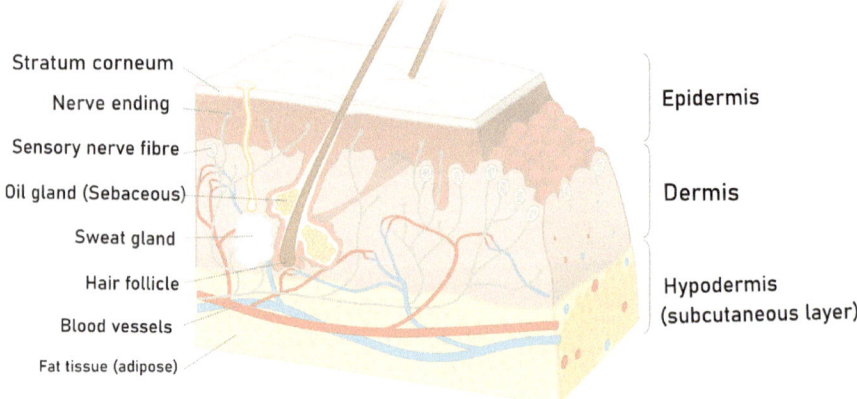

Fig. 3.1 Skin anatomy

desmosomes, now fuse together to form the so-called "cornified envelope" and are continuously and imperceptibly exfoliated to the outside.

In addition to the epidermal keratinocytes, the epidermis contains the melanocytes responsible for pigmentation of the skin and the dendritic Langerhans cells with immunological function, located in the suprabasal layer.

The sensory function of the skin is also localized in the epidermis. Sensitive, free nerve endings extend into the stratum corneum and mediate pain, temperature stimuli, and surface sensitivity. Meissner's tactile corpuscles and Merkel's nerve endings can be found in the basal epidermis, along with (somewhat deeper) Vater Paccini corpuscles. Together, they mediate so-called depth sensitivity such as pressure, stretch, and vibration (Fig. 3.2).

3.2.2 The Dermis

The human dermis is only loosely interspersed with connective tissue cells (fibroblasts) and consists essentially of a water-storing, partly amorphous, partly fibrillar extracellular matrix and vessels. Papillary and reticular dermis are distinguished by the density of the vascular network. In the papillary dermis, there is an extremely dense network of arteriovenous anastomoses (capillary loops) that protrude into the epidermis in the form of cones, thus allowing nourishment of the non-capillarized outer envelope (Fig. 3.1). The papillary dermis is also interspersed with numerous, open lymphatic fissures [1, 2].

3.2.3 The Reticular Dermis and Subcutis

The reticular dermis is traversed by larger afferent blood vessels and lymphatic channels and usually merges diffusely with the subcutaneous adipose tissue. The hair follicles, sebaceous glands, and sweat glands are located in this zone. The lymph nodes belonging to the skin are found in the subcutis (Fig. 3.1).

This is already illustrated by the threefold structure of the skin (Fig. 3.1). In the deep layers (hair papillae, sebaceous glands, and subcutaneous adipose tissue), proliferation and metabolic processes predominate, without a sharp boundary being able to be drawn between the lower dermis and the subcutis. The upper dermis is the site of rhythmic circulation. Here the blood circulation floods in the periphery and comes to reversal. In the zone of capillary anastomoses, cellular migration from capillaries to epidermis and back takes place. In the epidermis, proliferation is highly regulated and reduced to a few basal and follicle-associated stem cells. Towards the periphery, a strictly regulated death process (apoptosis) then occurs in the upper third of the epidermis as part of the terminal differentiation of the keratinocytes.

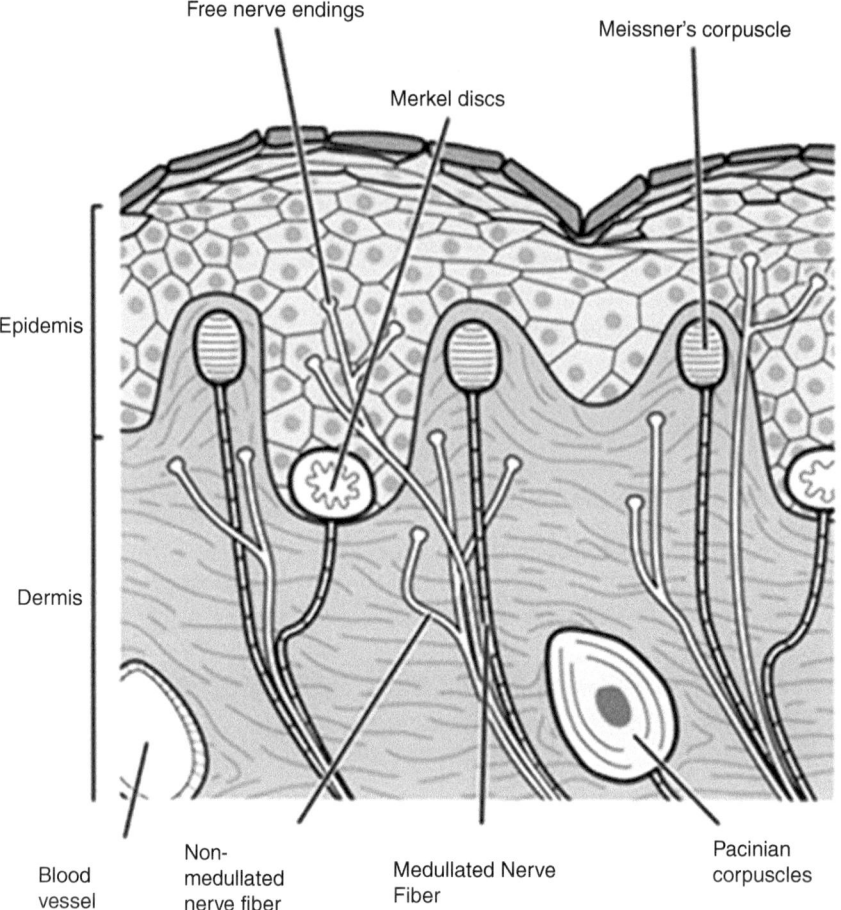

Free nerve endings

Meissner's corpuscle

Merkel discs

Epidemis

Dermis

Blood vessel

Non-medullated nerve fiber

Medullated Nerve Fiber

Pacinian corpuscles

Fig. 3.2 Skin nerve system

3.2.4 Tripartite Structure of the Human Skin-Associated Immune System

The immune system of the skin (skin immune system = SIS, skin associated lymphoid tissue = SALT) [3] can also be informally classified in the tripartite structure of the skin (Fig. 3.3).

In the epidermis, cellular elements dominate and serve mostly a detection purpose. While the keratinocytes migrate continuously from the basal layer to the outer border of the organism in the form of a continuous stream outward within 28 days, the epidermal Langerhans cells, as the "outermost sentinels of the immune system", hold their position in the suprabasal layer where they scan their surroundings for antigens or so-called danger signals. However, the melanocytes located underneath

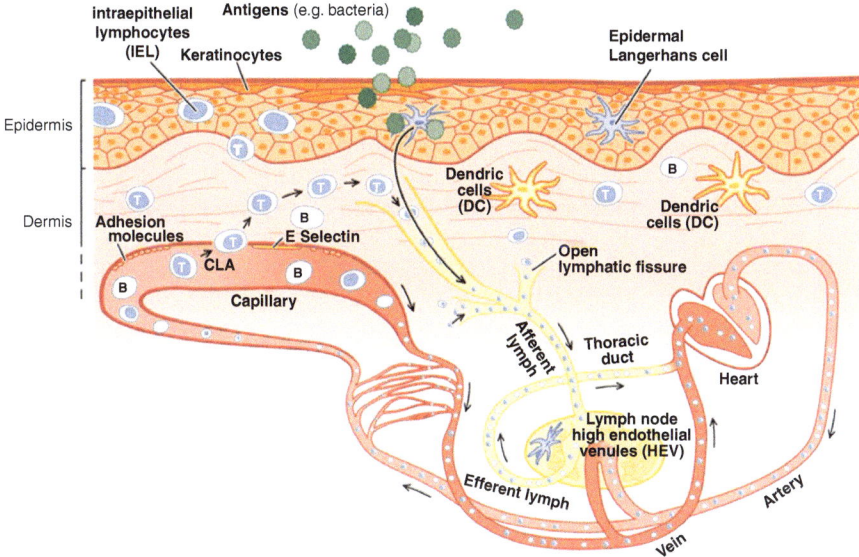

Fig. 3.3 Immunology of the skin

on the basal membrane also have a detection purpose, namely, for the sunlight hitting the skin from the outside. The concentration of sensory functions in this zone (free nerve endings in the epidermis, Merkel cells and Meissner bodies located in the cones of the papillary dermis) also matches the immunological detection function of the epidermis.

A lively exchange takes place between the skin and the blood system via the capillary system of the papillary dermis. Skin-specific, immunocompetent cells, predominantly lymphocytes, leave the capillaries in this zone, migrate as intraepithelial lymphocytes through the epidermis and leave the skin again via the efferent lymphatic channels. In case of danger signals, the Langerhans cells are activated, migrate out of the epidermis and leave the skin via the lymphatic pathways. On their way to the skin-associated lymph nodes, the Langerhans cells up-regulate their immunocompetence. Antigen presentation, cell activation, and proliferation of antigen-specific lymphocytes occur predominantly in the skin-associated lymph nodes. Immigration of specific and non-specific effector cells into the skin then occurs again via the circulation and capillary network of the dermis [3]. Thus, a clear spatial separation of detection, circulation, and proliferation can be seen in the skin-associated immune system (Fig. 3.3):

At the outermost boundary of the skin with the outside world, a cellular detective expression of the immune system predominates. The middle layers of the dermis are dominated by a dense capillary vascular network, which mediates the circulation and migration of immune cells. In the deeper layers of the skin, proliferative processes predominate.

3.3   The Development of Skin and Sense of Touch

During human embryogenesis, the amnion takes over the insulating and protective function of the skin for the embryo until the third trimester. It is not until the 24th week of pregnancy that the skin gradually becomes impermeable to water (Fig. 3.4).

Already in a 16-day-old human germinal vesicle, a division of the germinal disc into the ectoderm on the side facing the amnion cavity, the endoderm on the side facing the yolk sac, and the formation of the intermediate mesoderm is clearly visible (Fig. 3.4). After the folding of the neural tube and formation of the somites, a primitive two-layered epidermis is detectable after about 5 weeks, which rests on a simple basal membrane. The periderm is pluripotent, i.e., all cells can be divided indefinitely [4]. Later cell divisions in the epidermis are restricted to the stem cells of the stratum basale. After the eighth week, an intermediate layer is detectable between the periderm and the basal membrane, and shortly before that the boundary between the still cell-rich dermal tissue and the subcutis is also marked. At about the same time, the tooth systems, nail systems, and eccrine sweat glands are formed. From the tenth week on, the hair follicle and sebaceous gland anlagen follow and a multi-layered stratification of the epidermis occurs. The highly complex junctional zone between the epidermis and dermis with its various anchoring fibrils forms, and the superficial and deep vascular plexus develops in the dermis from the tenth week. Around the twelfth week, the so-called epidermal symbionts, the melanocytes, Langerhans cells, and Merkel cells migrate into the epidermis. At about the same period, the ingrowth of sensitive nerve fibers into the epidermis occurs, which branch in the stratum granulosum. Thus, organogenesis of the skin is completed

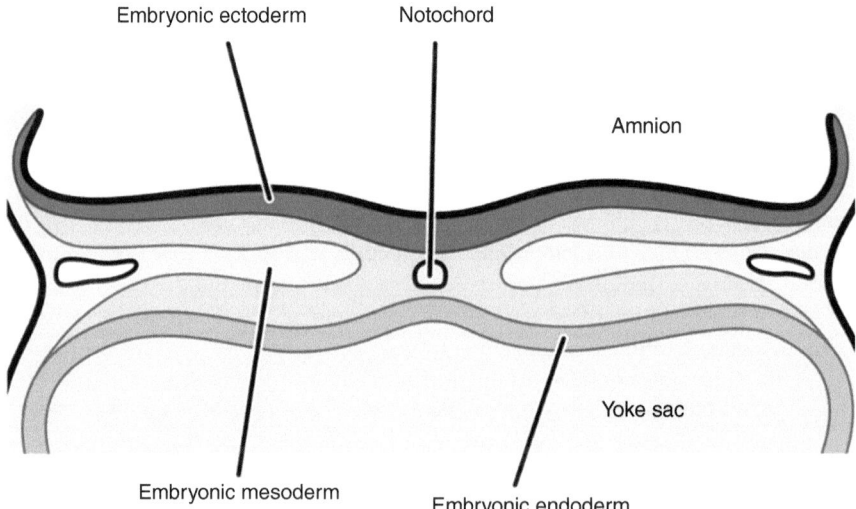

Fig. 3.4 Embryogenisis

toward the end of the first trimester [1, 4]. The sensory functions of the skin, including the sense of touch, is also fully developed at this time.

In the second trimester, the boundary between papillary and reticular dermis is formed and an undulating interlocking between epidermis and dermis (reteleistae) occurs. Keratinization now begins in the epidermis, initially at the hair follicles. Towards the end of the second trimester, the periderm is shed. Only at the beginning of the third trimester does the final formation of the multilayered epidermis with the basal layer, the prickle cell layer, the granular cell layer, and the horny layer occur. Interfollicular keratinization now reaches its completion. In the third trimester, vascular development also progresses in the skin. Capillary loops first develop palmar and plantar. On the rest of the skin, capillary loops do not develop until several weeks postnatally [1].

Thus, in a broad outline, human skin passes through stages of phylogenesis during ontogeny: first, a single-layered, pluripotent epidermis is present (stage of primitive metazoans), followed by a multilayered, nonkeratinized epidermis with epidermal symbionts of mesenchymal and neuroectodermal origin (stage of jawless and amphibian chordates), followed by a multilayered, keratinized squamous epithelium (detectable from terrestrial amphibians onward). In contrast to reptiles and birds, in humans there is no reduction of glands and excessive keratinization, the thin state of the epidermis present at birth with only slight keratinization remains throughout life [5].

3.4 Characteristics of Children's Skin—Implications for External Applications

Children's skin differs from adult skin in many respects. It makes up a significantly larger proportion in relation to body weight and is up to 30% thinner than that of adults. As a result, children's skin offers less protection, is more sensitive, and reacts more quickly and intensively to external influences.

Due to the structure of the skin itself, as well as the ongoing physical and psychological development children are undergoing, external applications on children should be carried out with extra care. In the case of newborns and infants, some factors should be particularly taken into account and applications should be adjusted accordingly. Special attention should be paid to the duration of the application, the quality and dosage of the substances used and the temperature of the application. But also the quality of the associated touch has a much greater role than in adults.

At birth, the horny layer of infant skin is about 30% thinner than that of adults, thus the skin loses fluid more quickly. Children have an increased sensitivity to stimuli such as touch and essential oils, which should therefore be diluted accordingly, with a neutral oil (depending on the concentration of the starting substance) as needed.

In infants and children, the subcutaneous fatty tissue is not yet fully developed, therefore the skin also reacts more sensitively to stimuli and cold. Due to the thinner subcutaneous fatty tissue, care must be taken to ensure that children are kept warm during treatment to protect them from hypothermia.

The sebaceous and sweat glands are not yet fully developed in infants and the sebaceous glands produce few lipids, so that there is not yet a sufficiently protective greasy film on the skin. Their pH value is still neutral in the first days after birth. Due to the reduced sweating, newborns cannot yet fully regulate their body temperature. This also means that absorption through the skin is faster, and only high-quality substances should be used.

The ratio of skin surface to body weight is about 2–3 times greater in infants than in adults, which means that the skin loses fluid more quickly and provides a larger surface for bacteria and fungi to attack. The anatomical structure means that a relatively large area is treated when applying to children and the effect of an application can be very intense. Therefore, it is particularly important to maintain rather gentle temperature differences between the body temperature and an application (bath, tea, and oil applications).

This is especially true for premature infants whose skin, depending on the gestational age, has hardly any barrier function—which is why they are cared for in an appropriately moist and warm environment of an incubator. When appropriate attention is given to external factors (especially warmth!) premature infants can also spend many hours in direct skin-to-skin contact with a parent, which is extraordinarily useful for early bonding. As already mentioned, the quality of touch plays an extremely important role. Taking into consideration all these factors does not mean that premature babies should not receive external applications. However, these should be carried out exclusively by people who are experienced and specifically trained (in individual cases, this can also be the parents).

References

1. Bolognia JL, Jorizzo JL, Rapini RP (2003) Dermatology. Mosby, Edinburgh, pp 23–84
2. Fritsch P, Schwarz T (2018) Dermatologie und Venerologie. In: Grundlagen, klinik, atlas. 3. Auflage. Springer, Berlin
3. Bos JD (2003) Skin immune system. In: Cutaneous immunology and clinical immunodermatology. CRC Press, Boca Raton
4. Christ B (1993) Entwicklung der Haut. In: Hinrichsen KV (ed) Human-embryologie. Springer, Berlin, pp 863–870
5. Schempp CM, Emde M, Wölfle U (2009) Dermatologie im Darwinjahr: Die Evolution der Haut. JDDG 7:750–757

Therapeutic Effects of External Applications

4

Matthias Bertram

4.1 Do External Applications Work?

Effectiveness is an important keyword to begin this discussion. In a sense, it marks the divide where the differences between more scientifically-oriented acute medical treatment and more unconventional therapeutic directions are revealed. Take the case of sleep disorders. Various chemical drugs are available, among them benzodiazepines, which can be resorted to in severe cases. The desired *effect* is sleep (physiological effect). However, the *side effects* can be serious. This treatment acts on the symptom of insomnia; while the underlying sleep disorder often remains untreated.

Effectiveness, on the other hand, can also be used to describe the therapeutic benefit for a specific person in their particular life and illness situation. Applied 'Rhythmic Embrocation According to Wegman/Hauschka', for example, can be *effective* in helping a patient suffering from severe tumor pain to *sleep comfortably for a while* ([1], p. 180). Gerhard Kienle, the German anthroposophical doctor, neurologist, health politician and scientific theorist referred to this distinction in meaning with revision of the German Medicines Act, a law passed to regulate medicinal products in Germany, as early as the 1970s: not only changes in isolated physiological parameters can be used to evaluate a treatment, but rather the overall therapeutic effect is decisive [2].

M. Bertram (✉)
Doerthe-Krause-Institute for Nursing Science and Education, Gemeinschaftskrankenhaus Herdecke gGmbH, Herdecke, Germany
e-mail: m.bertram@gemeinschaftskrankenhaus.de

In scientific medical research, the controlled clinical trial is the dominant standard. The aim is to statistically test therapeutic interventions under standardized conditions. If the (measured) results in the study group are significantly better than those in the control group, which received a different intervention or a placebo, the intervention is interpreted as effective. This conclusion is based on the scientific logic that the intervention can be interpreted as the *cause of* physiological processes—much like how increasing the temperature of water on a stove top must necessarily cause the water to boil and evaporate when it reaches a certain level.

According to this logic, every person should respond in the same way to a standardized intervention. However, as therapists know, this is not the case. *Organisms,* unlike *mechanisms,* respond uniquely, *interpreting* the therapeutic stimulus in their own individual way. Chilean biologists and philosophers Humberto Maturana and Francisco Varela created the concept of *autopoiesis* in the 1980s to understand biological systems [3]. Autopoiesis means self-generation, a system capable of reproducing and maintaining itself. The essence of organisms is characterized by the fact that their physiology is not externally controlled, but follows rules that are intrinsic to them, in a sense 'they cause themselves'. A stimulus from the environment—even if it is therapeutic—can therefore never be the cause of a reaction, it can only be the *trigger* for the organism's own (healing) processes ([1], pp. 52–54).

This fundamental insight, that a living relationship exists between organisms and their environment, is at least 200 years old. The natural scientist Alexander von Humboldt identified the connection between his botanical research objects and their environment early on in an intensive exchange with the poet and scientist Johann von Goethe, and natural philosopher Friedrich Schelling, and other intellectual giants of his time.

First, he took up the concept of *organism* in his investigations, concluding that while in a mechanical system the parts form the whole, in an organic system, the whole forms the parts ([4], p. 55). Later, he made comparisons between plants from different parts of the world and in different climates. The results were incorporated into his famous nature paintings. These complex graphics are carefully and empirically displayed evidence of the rigid connection between organisms and their environments. He summarized his thoughts in the paper *Ideas for a Geography of Plants*: (Ibid, p. 171). The similarity of plants, he argues, does not depend on their geographical location but rather on climatically similar conditions.

Immanuel Kant had previously limited Western thinking to a consciousness that is enclosed in the brain. According to him, the mind can only use its sensory experiences to analytically dissect the world and speculate about the connection of the parts. How it *really is* remains hidden from it ([5], p. 13). Humboldt, on the other hand, recognized nature as a living organism, in which everything is related to everything else and is mutually dependent. Thus, as early as 1800, he was able to name and explain the connection between the deforestation of the rainforests he observed and the changes in climate ([4], p. 86). Herein lies the origin of the ecology movement. Since Humboldt, Goethe, and the philosopher and theologian Johann Gottfried Herder, and others, the world can be thought of ecologically, as an interconnection between the whole and its parts.

This ecological interconnection, which also exists between a human being and their (therapeutic) environment, also provides a rich area for integrative medicine. Central to this approach is the concept of the body. "In phenomenology, a distinction is made between the body, which is our *lived body*, through which we experience, feel and move, and the *physical body*, which is a mere object and can accordingly be called a 'body thing'" ([6], p. 15). The *lived body* is an entity through which we are subjectively connected and which allows us to be perceptive and active in the world. This becomes clear, for example, in pain, which is not *had* by "the body out there" but rather experienced by the subject themselves, "I have pain."

In contrast, ones connectedness with the world (nature) can also be experienced tangibly when taking action (e.g., peeling potatoes, driving a car, drawing blood) not in the body itself (muscle spindles of the arms, tactile receptors of the fingers) but at the end of the tool (cutting edge of the knife, car tire on a rain-soaked road, tip of the cannula needle). In this way, tools become an extension of the lived body ([7], p.13). The subjectively experienced body is always already the lived body in its environment. By means of the lived body, a person is not passively in the world, but actively in the world, synchronizing with it. The philosopher of phenomenology, Edmund Husserl called this active state "lived embodiment" [8], the activities of which are initially unconscious or preconscious. The basic preconscious mode of the body is called *intentionality*. It is the key to understanding body phenomenology.

Independently of body phenomenology, the physician and philosopher Victor von Weizsäcker described this synchronization and called it a Gestalt circle [9]. This can be illustrated by the example of the sense of sight. If one pays attention to the eye movements of a person sitting opposite, who is looking out the window of a moving train, a peculiar phenomenon is noticeable. The observed person shows a nystagmus; the eyes always move slowly in one direction and then suddenly snap back to their starting point. This activity of the eye muscles is necessary to perceive the passing landscape. The eyes follow a fixed point in order to jerkily take a new point into view when the last one disappears from the field of vision. This means that the eye muscles act unconsciously in a sensory way to enable the perception of the landscape. And also, the receptors on the retina do not produce a passive image of the environment, but manipulate it actively in different ways (for example by edge contrast sharpening).

This example clearly shows, being perceptively active in an environment presupposes bodily activity. Muscles and receptors interact with each other and with their environment. They approach perception or, strictly speaking, precede it—an eye that 'knew' nothing about landscapes would stare straight ahead. Optical noise would be the consequence, only meaningful movement and "image processing" allow recognition. This mode of the body, its intentionality, reveals itself in this preconscious active and meaningful synchronization of a body with its environment. The two cannot be thought of without the other; they are rigidly coupled [10].

Integrative medicine addresses the senses in a variety of ways. Here, too, the bodily processes triggered by sensory stimuli reveal the meaningful bodily comprehension of the environment as an expression of intentional resonance. This is the basis of therapeutic effects—and an expression of the autopoiesis of the human organism. Even to disease stimuli (e.g., a rhinovirus) there is a meaningful reaction (by the swelling of the nasal mucous membranes, rise in temperature, increase of lymphocyte count, and other physiological processes). This part of bodily intentionality is called self-healing. It is an immanent (acting autopoietically) part of all organisms.

Experience from medical spas, for example, shows how effectively organisms react to stimuli from the environment by means of this capacity for meaningful bodily resonance. Both too low and too high blood pressure can be effectively treated by Kneipp cold water (hydrotherapy; cf. [11]). The organism reacts autopoietically; it "knows what to do" [12].

In the therapeutic stimulation of the self-healing powers through external applications, one sense takes a special position, the sense of touch. While the other senses lead consciousness out into the world, the sense of touch throws it back to the experience of one's own body ([13], p. 114). Strictly speaking, through the sense of touch, we initially feel nothing other than our physical outer limit. It conveys to us the perception that we bump up against something with our skin that is not identical to ourselves.

This experience is of elementary importance for the development of the human being. By being pressed through the birth canal, an infant experiences the loss of oneness with the world and an awakening to its separateness in it. It is through this experience of the boundary between self and world that consciousness emerges ([1], p. 181). The intentionality of the lived body is an uninterrupted centrifugally directed activity towards the world. Only in resistance does it come up against the limits that the world sets for the lived body and thereby awakens it. "... in its development into reflective self-consciousness, resistances gradually become objects" ([13], p. 114). To open up the world means to *grasp* it. In this way, first consciousness of the world arises, and in being thrown back onto oneself, finally self-consciousness arises.

Touch therefore has a special significance in a therapeutic setting. If it is to be healing, it requires attentiveness and experience. For nurses, therapists, and physicians, active touch is part of everyday life. It can provide orientation and save many words; it can convey confidence and hope; it can also simply create the certainty of not being alone. But touch is always intimate; it is easy for boundaries to be crossed.

Massages, therapeutic touch or Rhythmic Embrocation According to Wegman/Hauschka, can be highly effective therapeutic methods—if applied correctly. They are often the first choice for pain of the musculoskeletal system [14]. Here, too, it is a matter of offering the sick body the right stimuli to trigger the right self-healing processes. Pain is not simply anesthetized, rather, its character is changed—the person is no longer defenselessly plagued by their pain, they regain agency over it. They can, for example, characterize their pain more precisely, localize it, identify links to times of day, and exposure to hot/cold stimuli. This pain *transformation* is an important prerequisite for further targeted interventions ([1, 15], p. 17–18).

In most people, a Rhythmic Embrocation According to Wegman/Hauschka (RhE) leads to a phenomenon which we have called *being uncaged*. This is the subjectively experienced liberation from stereotypes of bodily activity. This can concern the locomotor system as well as emotions, thoughts, the ways of communicating, and self-perception.

Patients suffering from anorexia nervosa often react to RhE after several treatments with a relaxation of their entire musculoskeletal system that was previously unknown to them. They no longer lie cramped on the treatment table. "These anorexics often have completely raised shoulders [...] And it often takes close to two months, until their shoulders can loosen a little more and even touch the table," said an expert for RhE ([1], p. 124). Many nurses know what a wonderful sleep aid an RhE can be. A patient with sleep disorders in the hospital reported, "You know, I can always hear everything that is outside; I can also tell by the step which on of you is walking past my door. ...But when I'm lying here and I'm getting an embrocation, I don't hear it at all." It's as if the patients are "retracting their antennas."

It is not uncommon for patients to burst into tears after an RhE. Although this is sometimes unpleasant for them, it is rarely an expression of suffering. Often, it is more a relief to have finally found themselves again. For example, after an RhE, a patient spoke of the death of her husband. In tears, she confessed that it was the first time in a long time that she had cried over this loss. Now, finally, to her great relief, she was able to grieve (Ibid, p.132). Other patients feel liberated from a long redundant protective posture after an operation; for still others, an RhE interrupts an agonizing compulsive flow of speech (Ibid, p. 130–131). Even thinking itself can become stuck in unproductive patterns. Thus, this disengagement from unconsciously habitual behavioral routines can also lead patients to feel surprisingly capable of making judgments and decisions—for example, for or against therapy (Ibid, p. 141–143).

As has been shown, other body-related therapies can also trigger these and similar reaction patterns. In the context of the present discussion, all these findings can be summarized with the statement: Any meaningful touch can stimulate the ability to come to oneself and to become capable of acting appropriately again. It does not occur in every case, but therapists should expect it. It is one of the ways in which the effects of external applications can be characterized. Their potential effectiveness can be grouped with other specialized therapy methods accompanied by attentive touch.

When evaluating the therapeutic potential of the methods described in this text, it is often claimed that the findings are subjective in nature, that they cannot be proven objectively. Objectivity itself is a quality criterion from scientific research. It is based on the aim of designing a study and achieving test results that are as independent as possible from the persons conducting the research. It is sometimes forgotten that the results of research are always ultimately evaluated by subjects.

Humans are no less complex than their biological environment, and diverse sciences are needed to deepen understanding. Scientific medicine, anthropology, medical sociology, psychology, milieu-therapeutic research [16], and others open different windows and dimensions under which the human being can be explored. An empirically working body phenomenology is one of these dimensions. In the tradition of Goethe and Humboldt, Husserl and philosopher and Christian mystic Jakob Boehme, it seeks to focus on the interconnection between humans and their environment. Here we are interested in which therapies (environmental factors) could trigger which healing processes.

Of course, lived body processes ultimately have physical effects as well. They can lower blood pressure, stimulate the immune system (increasing the lymphocyte count), or relieve stress (lowering cortisol levels). This is the large field of research for Mind-Body-Medicine, at least where it involves scientific research [12, 17, 18]. However, understanding which phenomena can be interpreted as effective requires other scientific approaches as well. Examples are the above-mentioned phenomena of *being able to sleep comfortably*, *being uncaged*, and *pain transformation*. Once the essence of these concepts is known, they become recognizable to therapists in the reactions of their patients. They take on diagnostic significance and it becomes understandable how they can enhance healing processes and improve quality of life.

References

1. Bertram M (2005) The therapeutic process as dialogue: structural-phenomenological investigation of rhythmic rubs according to Wegman, Hauschka. Pro Business, Berlin
2. Kienle G (1974) Drug safety and society: a critical examination. Schattauer, Stuttgart, New York
3. Maturana HR, Varela FJ (2009) The tree of knowledge: the biological roots of human cognition, vol 17855. Fischer-Taschenbuch-Verl, Frankfurt, M
4. Wulf A (2016) In: Kober H (ed) Alexander von Humboldt and the invention of nature. C. Bertelsmann, Munich
5. Waldenfels B (1992) Phenomenology. UTB S. UTB GmbH, Stuttgart
6. Waldenfels B (2000) The bodily self: lectures on the phenomenology of the body, vol 1472. Suhrkamp, Frankfurt am Main
7. Böhme G (2003) Leibsein als Aufgabe: Leibphilosophie in pragmatic terms. Zug, Switzerland, p 38
8. Husserl E, Ströker E (1995) Cartesian meditations: an introduction to phenomenology, vol 291, 3rd edn. Felix Meiner, Hamburg
9. Weizsäcker V v (1973) The gestalt circle: theory of the Unity of perceiving and moving. Frankfurt a. Main, Suhrkamp
10. Fuchs T (2013) The brain - a relational organ: a phenomenological-ecological conception, 4th edn. Kohlhammer, Stuttgart
11. Sandmann F-K (ed) (2017) Healing with the power of nature. Insel Verlag, Berlin
12. Bertram M, Kolbe H-J (eds) (2016) Dimensions of therapeutic processes in integrative medicine: an ecological model. Springer, Wiesbaden
13. Fuchs T (2000) Body, space, person: outline of a phenomenological anthropology. Klett-Cotta, Stuttgart
14. Lange U, Müller-Ladner U (2008) Evidence on physical medicine therapy options for musculoskeletal pain. Z Rheumatol 67(8):658–664
15. Bertram M (2003) The therapeutic process as dialogue. Methodological considerations and methodological strategies for researching nursing-therapeutic processes. In: Matthiessen PF, Ostermann T (eds) Individual case research in medicine: meaning, possibilities, limitations. University of Witten, Herdecke, pp 104–134

16. Kramer M (2016) Designing therapeutic settings. In: Bertram M, Kolbe H-J (eds) Dimensions of therapeutic processes in integrative medicine: an ecological model. Springer, Wiesbaden, pp 231–246
17. Rüegg JC (2012) Mind & body: how our brain influences health. Knowledge & life. Schattauer, Stuttgart
18. Storch M, Cantieni B, Hüther G, Tschacher W (eds) (2011) Embodiment: understanding and using the interaction of body and psyche; with supplementary chapter "embodiment in the Zurich resource model (CRM)", 2nd edn. Huber, Bern

Techniques: Instructions for External Applications

Kira Bindewald

This chapter describes techniques of various external applications that can be used on pediatric patients. It provides concrete instructions for their implementation, including descriptions, lists of materials needed, and illustrations to help the reader understand and apply each technique. All external applications included are suitable for children over the age of 1 year; applications suitable for infants are described in a separate sub-section (see Sect. 5.4).

The implementation of external applications for pediatric patients requires some special adjustments. For example, unlike when working on adult patients, it can be helpful to a pediatric patient to have a trusted person present; applications should not last too long; and it is ok to speak during an application, if this is soothing for the patient [1].

Often, a special calmness develops in the room during an application. To achieve this desired atmosphere, the applications should be carried out carefully, as described. In addition, when the application is a rhythmic embrocation, there are three pillars of elementary importance for the correct learning of the technique [1, 2]:

- The observation of a rhythmic embrocation by someone who has mastered the technique.
- The performance of a rhythmic embrocation under practical guidance and
- Experiencing a rhythmic embrocation on one's own body.

K. Bindewald (✉)
Integrative Medicine in Pediatric Oncology, Department of Pediatric Oncology and Hematology Charité, Universitätsmedizin Berlin, Berlin, Germany
e-mail: Kira.Bindewald@charite.de

5.1   Steps of an External Application

- Indication
- Application planning
- Preparation
- Implementation
- Post-treatment rest
- Evaluation

Note Before beginning any treatment, clarify whether the application you have selected is classified as medical care and therefore requires a physician's prescription. This will differ in each country, depending on the legal situation and the medical environment. If the planned application is considered a part of basic care, nursing staff can generally order and perform it under their own authority.

5.1.1   Indication

In order to set up a framework for an external application, begin by asking the patient whether they already have any experience with external applications. Identify the symptoms and state an indication to help define the treatment goal. In a preliminary interview, ask the patient to describe their complaints and expectations of a treatment. When working with young children, it may be necessary to have a trusted person (e.g., parent) present who can help describe the symptoms and, if needed, remain in the room while the application is being performed [3].

5.1.2   Application Planning

Using the information gathered from the patient, plan the application. Decide which body area will be treated, which techniques will be used, and which substance/s will be applied.

Give the patient and their trusted person information about how the application will proceed, including the duration, the patient's position during the application, as well as how any selected substance may feel (consistency, temperature…) when applied [1].

5.1.3   Preparation

Prepare the substance/s to be used and have all the required materials at the ready. Prepare the environment by ventilating the application room beforehand, adjusting the room temperature, and preparing the place where the patient will be seated or lying (chair, couch, bed…). It is also important to ensure quiet and privacy; if possible, hang a sign on the door.

5.1.4 Implementation

Perform the external application on the patient. This is the stage where you have physical contact with the patient through massaging, washing, or applying a compress. Take the time to consider the environment; the positioning of the patient and yourself; the sequence of the application; its duration; and, if applicable, the number of repetitions that will be needed. The presence of an assistant or a person trusted by the patient can be useful and, in some circumstances, is obligatory [3].

5.1.5 Post-Treatment Rest

The full effects of the external application can only be achieved through a combination of the treatment and the post-treatment rest period. Following an application, the patient should rest for 15–30 min. To allow the patient to fully relax, ensure they are comfortable and warm. If necessary, cover them with a blanket or large towel. After a rhythmic embrocation, the area treated should be wrapped before the rest period begins [2].

When working with an infant or toddler, it may be difficult for them to stay still and they should not be forcibly restrained. In this case, look for a quiet and calm activity such as looking at a book together [4].

5.1.6 Feedback Evaluation

Following the post-treatment rest period, or later in the day, do an feedback evaluation with the patient and/or their trusted person [1]. This should address how the application felt, what was pleasant/unpleasant, and what effects may have resulted. Since pediatric patients are not always able to verbalize consciously, the patient's spontaneous reactions during the application can also be considered feedback in the evaluation.

5.2 Effects of External Applications

The therapeutic challenge is to find the right application and the right substance for each patient. Each technique has a different effect on a patient's body and psyche [1]. For a conceptual framework and effective factors of external applications, see Chap. 2. A discussion of the therapeutic effects of external applications can be found in Chap. 4.

A broad division can be made between more calming and more activating external applications. A rhythmic embrocation can have either an activating or calming effect depending on the active quality of the touch; temperature of the application; the pace and the intensity of pressure applied during the treatment. Both embrocations and warm compresses can be used to help a patient relax and enhance their circulation, by removing lymphatic fluid from an affected part of the body and increasing the supply of oxygen to the tissues. Warm compresses have an additional calming effect due to the passive and local application of heat [3].

By contrast, hot compresses and those using intensely warming substances such as mustard or ginger, can be used to give a strong short-term stimulating effect and promote blood circulation. Cold compresses can also be used to stimulate circulation, by causing temporary vasoconstriction followed by vasodilation. This triggers hyperemia and thus leads to muscle relaxation. Cold compresses are therefore suitable for the treatment of acute pain and inflammation as well as acute sprains [3].

Another aspect of external applications is how they support the body in its own healing process. For example, fever is a symptom of overcoming an infection and thus part of the body's own defense reaction. External applications such as washes or calf wraps, do not seek to suppress the fever itself, but to combat the stressful accompanying symptoms such as circulatory instability, headache, or pain in the limbs [1, 3].

In general, external applications can invoke a sense of calm in patients. The caring attention they receive contributes to a sense of security and well-being, and an overall positive therapy experience.

Contraindications of external applications should be assessed in each individual case. In general, caution should be taken around existing inflammatory processes, defective skin areas, sensitive skin, e.g., due to chemotherapy, in tumor areas and in the presence of fever. In addition, an application should not be carried out with a substance that the patient finds unpleasant [2].

When using external applications, remember:

- The application should be discontinued if the patient finds it or the substance used to be unpleasant; if the patient feels uncomfortable during the treatment; or if the patient wishes it at any moment.
- The patient should always be in a comfortable position; if necessary, support should be provided with positioning materials.
- The patient should always be dressed warmly or covered to prevent them from cooling. Only the area to be treated should be exposed and then subsequently covered with a cloth.
- The room should be at a comfortable temperature and quiet, the patient should feel at ease.
- Depending on the patient's wishes, trusted persons can be present or even involved in the application itself.

5.3 Rhythmic Embrocation

Rhythmic embrocation originated at the beginning of the twentieth century, based on the rhythmic massage techniques of Dr. Ita Wegman. These were further developed by Dr. Margarethe Hauschka into a teachable concept, especially for therapists and nurses. The embrocations included in this book have been modified and do not bear the official designation of "Rhythmic Embrocation According to Wegman/Hauschka [1]."

At the end of the twentieth century, rhythmic embrocation became a fixed therapeutic component of nursing care, in institutions with an anthroposophic background. Rhythmic embrocations can be used in acute situations as well as for rehabilitation or prophylaxis. Thus, they can be practiced in almost all areas of clinical practice. The aim is to support the patient in their ability for self-healing and to rebalance a disturbed equilibrium [2].

During a rhythmic embrocation, in contrast to rhythmic massages, only gentle, mostly circular and, as the name suggests, rhythmic touches take place. The effect spreads over the entire body, similar to waves in water. Practitioners alternate between an emphasized touch (*binding*) and a lightness of touch (*loosening*), to create rhythmic impulses. The goal of which is to reestablish balance within and throughout the different parts of a patient's body, supporting natural healing processes. Through this approach, even the specific method of applying substances (in the form of oils or creams) is designed to increase their effect [1, 2].

The patient's body can be treated, either with a partial or a whole-body embrocation. Specialized embrocations of individual organs such as liver, spleen, or kidney, are advanced techniques and are not included in this book.

5.3.1 Procedure and Technique

During a rhythmic embrocation, it is important to be fully present and attentive while maintaining an unbiased and open-mind towards the patient. Your intention should be to support the healing and equilibrium of your patient to the very best of your ability. This means maintaining a state of inner calm, regardless of your own personal mood or sensitivities in the moment. The ability to observe the patient more attentively and to perceive any reactions they might experience to the application are increased with a calm demeanor. Ideally, performing a rhythmic embrocation should not be an exhausting activity and enables you to emerge from the application in a balanced state [2].

The quality of the touch is important during a rhythmic embrocation. Use the entire palm of your hand to create an enveloping effect and give a warming quality to your touch. Your hand should be relaxed; if the wrist is overstretched or your fingers are lifted, the muscles at the wrist and heel of your hand will tense up and harden—and the patient will notice. Rhythmic embrocation is done without pressure, tissue is worked without significantly moving or deforming it. The massage gestures are characterized by rhythmic flowing movements, during which the touch alternates between an emphasized touch (*binding*) and a light touch (*loosening*), to create rhythmic impulses. It can be helpful to try out the different intensities of touch on yourself to practice the gestures [1].

Always use an oil when implementing a rhythmic embrocation. This ensures the movements flow more easily; increases the warming effect; and allows for a substance effect, based on the type of essential oil used. If the patient is very sensitive to essential oils or finds them unpleasant, you can use a neutral oil instead [1].

Rhythmic embrocation on infants requires special considerations and techniques which are described in a special subsection of this chapter (see Sect. 5.4).

In order to successfully achieve the calming atmosphere desired during an application, it is important to carefully study and carry out the techniques as described. To truly learn the technique of rhythmic embrocation, practical hands-on instruction by someone who has mastered this technique is essential [2].

5.3.2   Materials Required

In addition to the hands of the practitioner, some materials are needed to perform a rhythmic embrocation [3].

- Support structure: couch, bed, or similar at working height.
- Positioning materials to enable a comfortable position for patient: knee bolster roll, (positioning) pillows, blankets, stools (to support the feet during a sitting position), etc.
- Blankets to cover the exposed areas of the body that are not being treated.
- Cotton cloths for wrapping the application area, e.g., muslin cloths, hand towels.
- Selected substance: neutral vegetable oil (base oil), e.g., almond, olive, or sunflower oil with the added essential oils, depending on the indication, or.
- A neutral vegetable oil (base oil) without added essential oils.
- Hot water bottle to warming the hands, if necessary.

5.3.3   Forehead Embrocation

- *Effects*: clarifying, invigorating, strengthening.
- *Indications*: headaches, mental exhaustion, physical disabilities.
- *Patient Position*: supine.
- *Practitioner Position*: standing at the head end of the patient.
- *Note*: either sect. 1 + 2 OR 1 + 3 is performed.

1. Place fingertips one after the other (first the index fingers and lastly the little fingers) in the middle of the forehead, above the eyebrows. From the starting point, rub in a circular shape. Move slowly downward and then outward toward the temples, emphasize the lower semicircle (downward and outward) and then complete the circle (upward and inward) with only very light contact. Your thumbs should not touch the patient's forehead.
2. Next, repeat the circle shape from the same starting point as described in Sect. 5.1, this time moving first upward towards the crown and then outwards toward the temples. Emphasize the outer movements along the temple only, using light touch for the rest of the circle. This creates a focusing, centering effect.
3. To achieve a widening, releasing effect, perform the circles as described in Sect. 5.2, moving first upwards to the crown, and outward toward the temples, but emphasize the entire upper semi-circle (upward and outward). During the upward movement, the tissue is pushed upward and then stretched outward (see Fig. 5.1).

5.3.4   Neck Tension Release

- *Effects*: releasing, warming, analgesic.
- *Indications*: (muscle) tension, neck pain, headaches.
- *Patient Position*: sitting/prone.
- *Practitioner Position*: behind the patient/standing to the side of the patient.
- *Note*: The spine itself should not be touched or crossed over.

The patient should lie on their stomach or sit covered in bed, with only their neck exposed. Place your fingertips from both hands simultaneously on either side of the

Fig. 5.1 Forehead embrocation

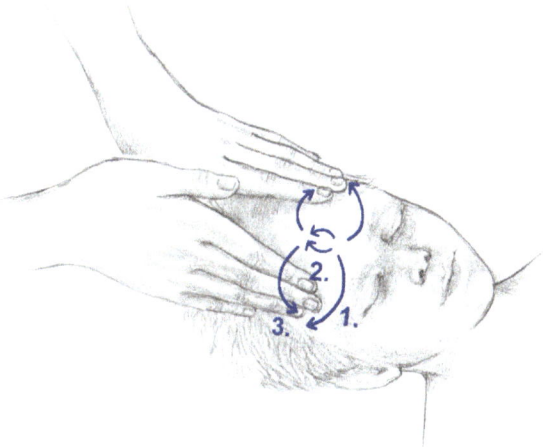

Fig. 5.2 Neck tension
release

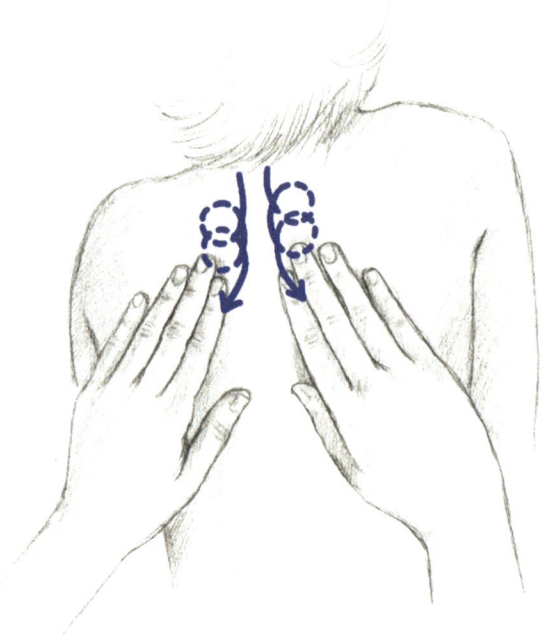

patient's spine with your fingertips pointing upward. Your thumbs should rest hori-
zontally (pointing inward) without actually touching the patient's spine, which
should remain contact-free during the entire application. The position of your hands
should create a triangle.

Begin with an emphasized touch as you bind the tissue from each side of the
spine toward the other; the tissue should form a small peak between your hands.
Slowly continue with this binding touch into a downward spiral shape. When the
spiral movement starts outward, loosen the tissue by slowly easing the pressure and
releasing between the thumb and fingers. Continue the spiral until your fingers
reach the underside of the patient's shoulder blade (see Fig. 5.2).

5.3.5 Shoulder Circles

- *Effects*: enveloping, releasing, calming, warming.
- *Indications*: (muscle) tension, shoulder pain.
- *Patient Position*: sitting/lateral position.
- *Practitioner Position*: standing sideways, facing the shoulder to be treated.

The patient should sit or lie on their side so that one shoulder is easily accessible.
Use both hands to envelop the shoulder, one hand from the front and the other from
the back.

Fig. 5.3 Shoulder circles

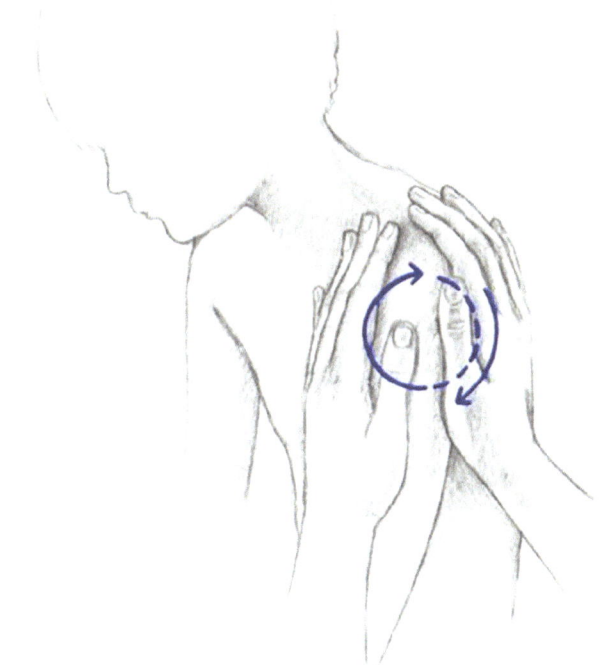

Now you will use both hands simultaneously, to make slightly different (staggered) clockwise circular motions.

Move your back hand in a downward semi-circle around the back of the shoulder joint. The entire movement is emphasized, binding the tissue which is only loosened as you gently lift your hand off the patient upon completion of the semi-circle.

Move your front hand in a full clockwise circle around the shoulder joint, without ever lifting contact with the skin. The tissue is bound through your emphasized upward movement and loosened as you complete the circle with a light touch.

After repeating several times, the movements are extended by enlarging the full circle made with the front hand to include the shoulder blade while your back hand traces the edge of the shoulder blade next to the spine, extending down to the level of the patient's posterior axillary line.

Finish the embrocation by using your front hand to make an accentuated downward stroke over the top of the shoulder to the shoulder blade. Finally, wrap the shoulder and repeat with the other shoulder (see Fig. 5.3).

5.3.6   Back Embrocation

There are several options for a back embrocation and each are described in detail below. A back embrocation always begins with applying oil, but depending on the patients' needs and the desired duration of the application, you may choose to do only one of the following options—or combine the One-Handed Circles with the Good Night Figure Eights. During a back embrocation, the patient can either sit or lie on their stomach/side.

Oil Application to the Back
- *Effects*: releasing, clarifying, creating structure.
- *Indications*: restlessness, obsessive thinking.
- *Patient Position*: sitting/prone/lateral position.
- *Practitioner Position*: behind the patient/standing to the side of the patient.
- *Note*: at the beginning of a back rub or as a single rub.

The first step of a back embrocation is to apply oil. This can be done with the patient in a sitting, prone, or lateral position.

Begin with one hand on each side of the patient's spine, gently dipping the heel of your hand, your palm, and then your fingers into the tissue at the nape of their neck. Slowly move your hands downward in straight lines (parallel to the spine), all the way to the beginning of the patients' buttocks. Lift, and begin again from the top but this time start from a little further toward the outside of the patient's body. Do again for a third time the same way, but starting from the posterior axillary downward. Repeat the entire sequence a maximum of three times (see Fig. 5.4).

Fig. 5.4 Oil application to the back

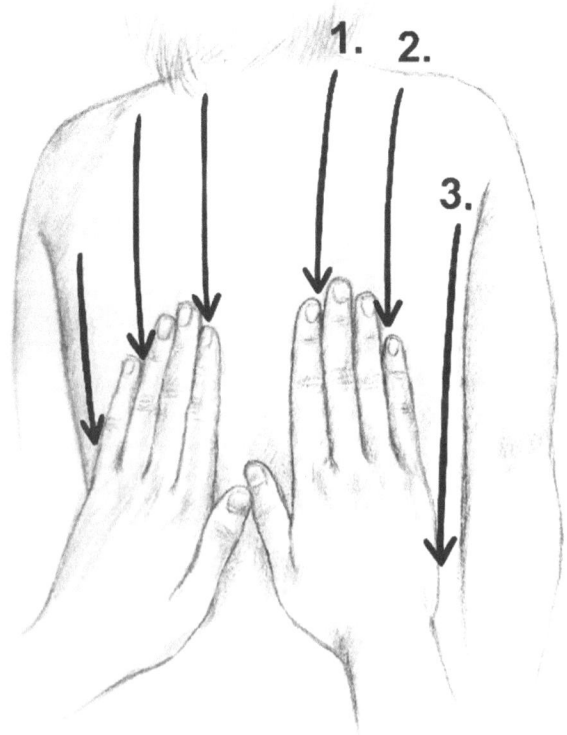

Figure Eights on the Back

- *Effects*: enveloping, balancing, harmonizing, warming.
- *Indications*: anxiety, restlessness, cold.
- *Patient Position*: prone/lateral/sitting.
- *Practitioner Position*: standing sideways to the patient.
- *Note*: Your active hand should remain parallel to the patient's shoulder line during the entire embrocation.

Once the back has been coated in oil, the figure eight rub can begin. Gently rest the hand closest to the patient on their shoulder. Use your other hand to gently dip down into the tissue on the outside at the far side of the patient's back, first with your fingers, and then with your palm and finally with the heel of your hand.

Move your hand as though it were drawing a horizontal figure eight across the entire width of the patient's back, continuously repeating this movement as you work your way down their back. The upper arc of each successive figure eight should overlap with the bottom arc of the previous one.

Emphasize the downward movements and bottom arcs of the figure eights to bind the tissue; and loosen by using a light touch on the upward movements and upper arcs of the figure eights. Your active hand should remain parallel to the shoulder line the entire time. Once you arrive at the patient's rump, come from the far side and make an emphasized downward stroke parallel to the spine. You can repeat or stop here. Cover the patient and then release your other hand from their shoulder (see Fig. 5.5).

One-Handed Back Circles

- *Effects*: structuring, uplifting, promotion of right-left perception.
- *Indications*: restlessness, slumped posture, hemiparesis.
- *Patient Position*: prone/lateral/sitting.

Fig. 5.5 Figure eights on the back

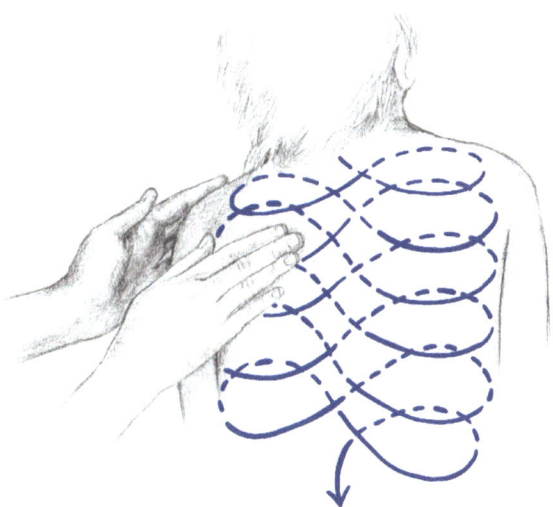

Fig. 5.6 One-handed back
circles

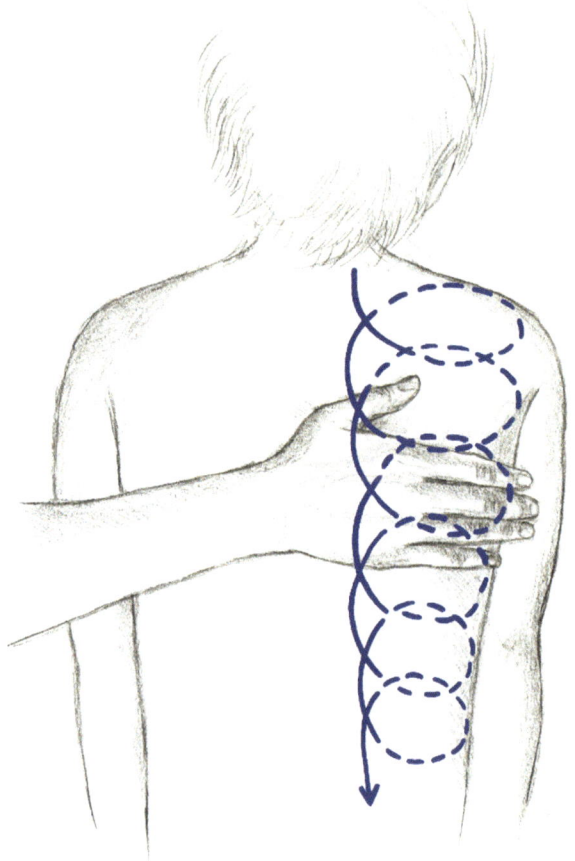

- *Practitioner Position*: behind the patient/standing to the side of the patient.
- *Note*: The area of the spine should not be left out of this application.

Begin by covering the untreated half of the back to prevent cooling. Rest your hand nearest to the patient on their shoulder. Gently dip the other hand into the tissue on the opposite side of the spine and begin a downward circular motion. Emphasize the downward movement next to the spine, binding the tissue before loosening it as you move upward to complete the circle with a light touch.

This circular motion continues downward like a spiral. Just as with the Figure Eight, the respective circles should slightly overlap. Use the ribcage to guide the active hand. To end, use an accentuated downward stroke along the spine before covering and doing the same on the opposite side of the back (see Fig. 5.6).

Good Night Figure Eights
- *Effects*: warming, calming.
- *Indications*: difficulty falling asleep, decubitus prophylaxis.
- *Patient Position*: prone/lateral/sitting.

- *Practitioner Position*: sideways to the patient/standing behind the patient.
- *Note*: If the upper arches are emphasized, kidney activity is stimulated.

The Good Night Figure Eights can be used to extend the One-Handed Back Circles, or each option can be used separately.

Follow the same procedure as described in the Figure Eights on the Back, but perform exclusively in the tailbone region. Take special care to form each figure eight evenly. This embrocation can be performed several times in succession.

5.3.7   Diamond Formation Embrocation

- *Effects*: mobilization of the diaphragm, deepened breathing, relaxation of the intestines.
- *Indications*: respiratory diseases, gastrointestinal diseases, meteorism, constipation.
- *Contraindications*: acute bleeding, ileus, appendicitis.
- *Patient Position*: supine.
- *Practitioner Position*: standing at the patient's pelvic level.
- *Note*: The Diamond Formation is also suitable for shock situations to activate breathing.

Gently press the heels of both your hands into the lower end of the sternum, with your fingers pointing outward to the sides. Slide both hands outward (in opposite directions), along the rib cage, toward the lumbar spine. When your fingertips reach the lumbar spine, lead with the heel of your hands as you trace the pelvic crest back to the patient's center. Gently ease the touch pressure and rest your hands here for a few seconds. Release touch with both hands simultaneously and repeat the application several times.

5.3.8   Two-Handed Abdominal Embrocation

- *Effects*: stimulates blood circulation, stimulates intestinal activity.
- *Indications*: meteorism, colic, constipation, postoperative dysfunction.
- *Contraindications*: unclear abdomen, ileus, appendicitis, acute hemorrhage.
- *Patient Position*: supine.
- *Practitioner Position*: standing sideways to the patient.

Using both hands, gently dip into the tissue directly to the right and left of the patient's belly button. Move your right hand in a semicircle, emphasizing the downward movement. Move your left hand in a complete circle around the belly button, emphasizing the sideways movements. Repeat the same formations with a slightly larger scale each time, expanding outwards to include the ascending colon, the transverse and descending colon. Use only finger tips to begin, but as the formations increase in size your whole palm should be in contact with the skin.

Fig. 5.7 Two-handed
abdominal embrocation

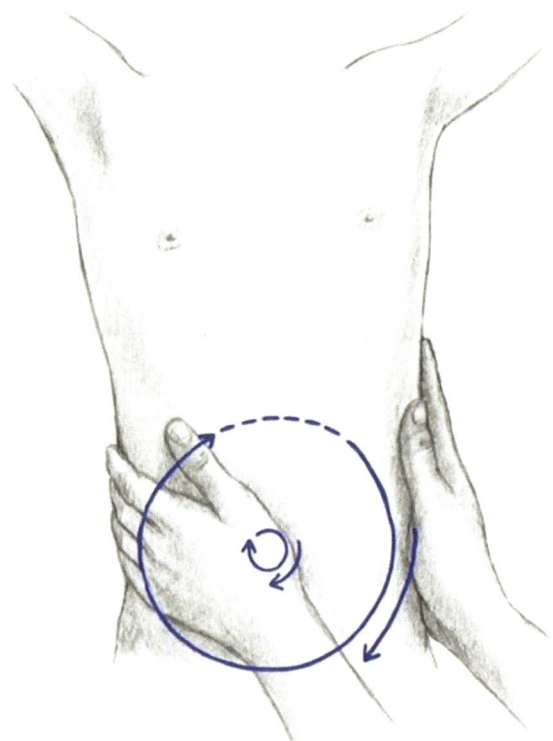

As the formations become larger, also take increasing care to lightly glide over the solar plexus, without actually losing skin contact.

End the embrocation by making an emphasized downward stroke with your right hand, starting from the left lower outer rib arch and following along the pelvic crest. Take extra care to stay along the pelvic crest so that there is no pressure placed on the bladder. Repeat this movement with your left hand, and then again for a final time with your right hand. Allow your right hand to linger briefly in its last position, while using your left to cover the patient's abdomen, then rest your left hand on the lower right pelvic arch. Now remove the right hand from its position and place along the lower left pelvic arch for a short moment. Remove both hands simultaneously (see Fig. 5.7).

5.3.9   Hand Embrocation

- *Effects*: releasing, soothing, warming.
- *Indications*: restlessness, anxiety, insomnia, cold hands, preactive stage of dying.
- *Patient Position*: sitting/supine.
- *Practitioner Position*: sitting slightly offset opposite the patient/standing to the side of the patient.

Fig. 5.8 Hand
embrocation

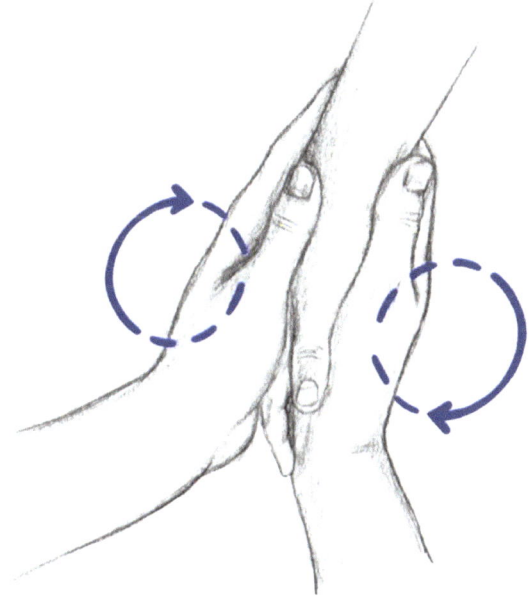

Sit opposite but slightly offset from the patient. Use a cushion to support the elbow of the hand to be treated, so that the patient can adopt a comfortable and relaxed posture.

Shape your hand furthest from the patient into a bowl-like form, into which the patient places their hand which is closest to you with the back of their hand facing your palm. Gently press the heel of your other hand into the patient's palm, enveloping the patient's hand between yours.

Begin to make (staggered) clockwise circles with both hands. The tissue is bound as you slightly increase the pressure whenever the heel of the hand closest to the patient, and the little finger of the other hand are directly opposite each other. When this meeting of the two passes, ease the pressure again.

After repeating several times, the treated hand is then covered and the process is repeated on the patient's other hand (see Fig. 5.8).

5.3.10 Figure Eights on the Fingers

- *Effects*: heightened awareness and agility, calming.
- *Indications*: spasms, hemiparesis, arthrosis, restlessness.
- *Patient Position*: supine/sitting/standing.
- *Practitioner Position*: standing sideways to the patient/sitting slightly offset opposite the patient.
- *Note*: Start with either the patient's thumb or index finger and continue to treat each finger in order until all have been treated.

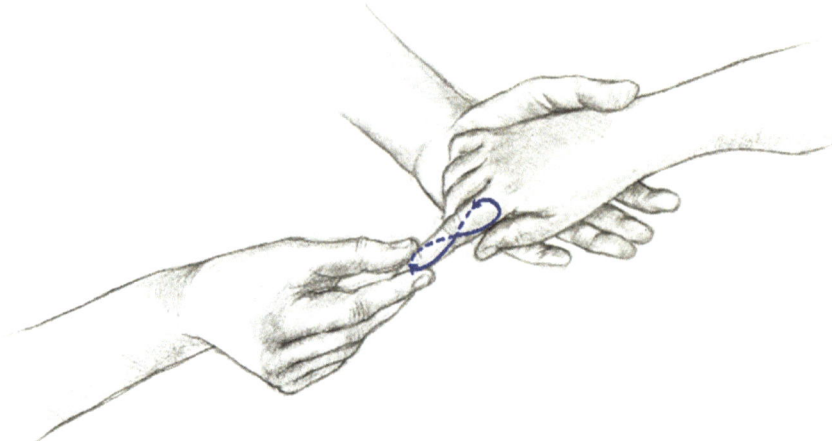

Fig. 5.9 Figure eights on the fingers

Sit opposite but slightly offset from the patient. Use a cushion to support the elbow of the hand to be treated, so the patient can adopt a comfortable and relaxed posture. Gently rest the patient's hand face down in the palm of your hand located furthest from the patient. Your palm should be touching theirs and be supporting their hand from below.

With your other hand, use your thumb and index finger to gently clasp both sides of the patient's index finger at the middle joint. Starting from this position, you will use your thumb and index finger to simultaneously trace parallel figure eights on opposite sides of their finger. To begin, move in the direction of their hand, in an upward semi-circle formation returning to the middle joint with a downward semi-circle, to complete a full circle. Now do the same movements in the direction of the fingertip, returning to the middle joint—simultaneously completing a horizontal figure eight on each side of the patient's finger.

Emphasize your movement from the middle joint toward the base joint. Once there, the light pressure is eased as you move back towards the middle joint. Increase emphasis once again as you move from the middle joint toward the fingertip, easing again from the fingertip back toward the middle joint.

To prevent the patient's finger from bending, you can use your middle or ring finger to lightly support it from below. After repeating several times, a final emphasized stroke is made from the middle joint to the fingertip to finish. Once all of the fingers on one hand have been treated, wrap the hand with an outer cloth (see Fig. 5.9).

5.3.11 Two-Handed Knee Circles

- *Effects*: warming, creating awareness.
- *Indications*: hemiparesis, knee pain.
- *Patient Position*: supine.

- *Practitioner Position*: standing sideways at the patient's knee level, facing toward the patient's head.
- *Note*: The hand closest to the patient circles clockwise around the right knee and counterclockwise around the left knee.

Expose the knee to be treated and, if necessary, support with a knee bolster roll or something similar so the patient is resting comfortably. Stand sideways at the patient's knee level, facing toward the patient's head.

Gently dip the hand nearest the patient into the inner side of their tibia, just below the knee. At the same time, gently press the other hand into the outside of their thigh, just above their knee joint. Use the hand below the knee, fully circle the patient's knee moving from the inside toward the outside. Use the other hand to make a semicircle on the outside of the leg, past the knee toward the calf. Once the semi-circle is complete, lift this hand and return it to its starting position.

Bind the tissue inward at the moment when both hands are opposite each other at knee height, the tissue should form a small peak between your hands. As you continue the movements, lighten your touch to loosen the tissue, much like when a handful of sand slowly trickles through the palm of the hand.

Repeat several times.

To end the embrocation, perform the same semicircular movement you have been doing, but this time using the other hand (one nearest the patient) with an emphasized stroke before lifting contact. Follow with a final emphasized semi- circle with the original hand (see Fig. 5.10).

5.3.12 One-Handed Calf Embrocation

- *Effects*: stimulates blood circulation, promotes feeling of lightness in heavy legs, warming.
- *Indications*: circulatory disorders, edema, muscle soreness.
- *Patient Position*: supine.
- *Practitioner Position*: standing sideways to the patient, facing the calf to be treated.

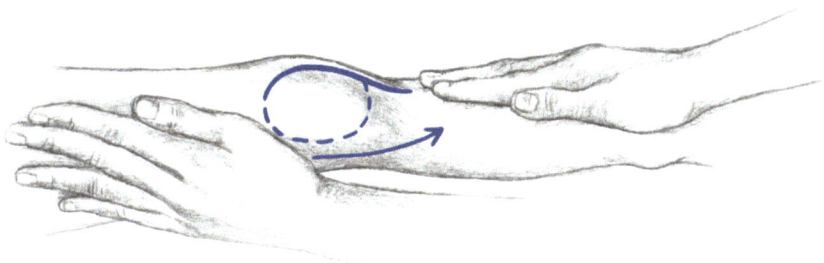

Fig. 5.10 Two-handed knee circles

The patient should lie on their back and be covered to keep warm. Place a support under their knees so that their calves are slightly elevated. Stand beside the patient facing towards their head. Lightly rest the hand located furthest from the patient to the outside of their knee.

With fingers leading, slide the other hand sideways around the leg to reach the patient's calf. Once there, turn the fingers so they are pointing upwards to the patient's head, their calf should now be resting comfortably in the palm of your hand.

Now press the palm of your hand slowly upwards until you have the feeling you are about to lift the leg. It is important that you push vertically upwards (towards the ceiling) and that there is no pressure in the direction of the head. Once the peak is reached, slowly release the tissue back down at the same tempo until you almost lose skin contact. As you gently slide your hand back to the inside of the calf, make a small forward circle so that you can repeat the movement pattern about a hand's width further down the calf without ever lifting contact.

As you move from the upper calf toward the foot, your hand should be increasingly horizontal. Continue until you reach the Achilles tendon. At the Achilles tendon, use only your fingertips. Finish the embrocation with an emphasized stroke on the inside next to the Achilles tendon, and over the heel (see Fig. 5.11).

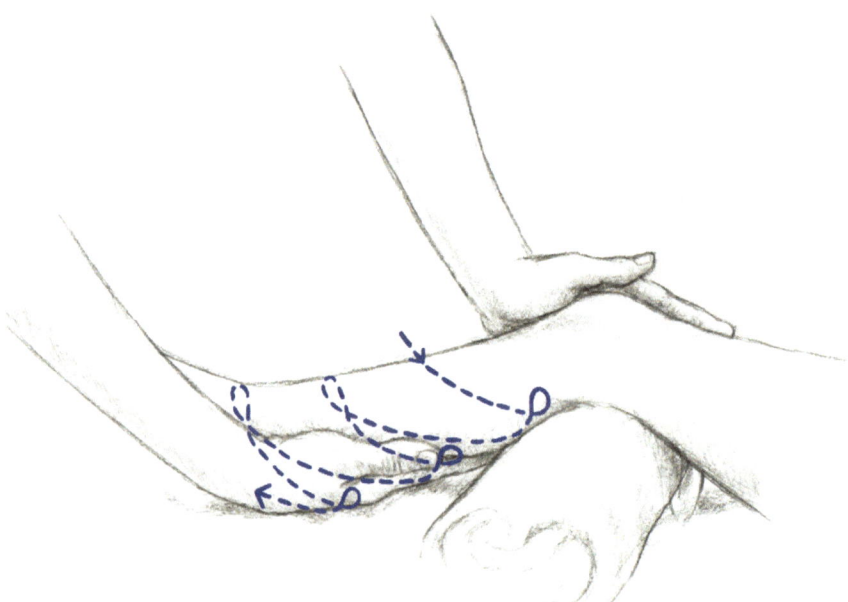

Fig. 5.11 One-handed calf embrocation

5.3.13 Foot Embrocation

- *Effects*: releasing, warming, calming.
- *Indications*: tension, restlessness, difficulty falling asleep, cold feet, headache, preactive stage of dying.
- *Patient Position*: supine/sitting.
- *Practitioner Position*: to the side of the patient, next to the foot about to be treated.
- *Note*: The following steps are meant to be performed one after the other, in the order listed.

Two-Handed Oil Application to the Foot
Use both hands to gently clasp the patient's foot from above and below. Your hand furthest from the patient should be on top and the other underneath their foot sole. Your thumbs should be placed along the inside of the foot, pointing upwards, parallel to the length of the foot. Your hands should be turned gently to form a V-shape between your thumbs and the other fingers.

Starting from the ankle joint and the arch of the foot, use both hands simultaneously to stroke the foot straight down to the toes. This wets the entire foot with oil and prepares it for the next steps. Repeat if the feet are particularly cold.

Two-Handed Foot Circles
After applying the oil as described above, leave your lower hand resting on the ball of the foot and toes. Lift your upper hand and return it back to its original starting position for the oil application. Once your upper hand is back in its original position, you can now lift your lower hand and return it to its original starting position. Do not remove both hands from the patient at the same time.

With both hands in their original position, you can now use them to slowly circle clockwise in the direction of the toes. Although you are using both hands at the same time, their circling should be staggered, i.e., as your upper hand is making a downward movement, your lower hand is making an upward movement. Emphasize the movement through the heel of your hand to the ball of your thumb.

As your circles reach the toes, lightly ease pressure by slightly opening and closing the hands for a light breathing movement. Return both hands to their original starting position one after the other. Repeat several times (see Fig. 5.12).

Heel Circles
After the Two-Handed Foot Circles, leave your lower hand under the ball of the foot, as you move your upper hand up above the heel to the area of the patient's Achilles tendon. Slightly lift the lower leg. Now you can remove the lower hand and use it to perform an emphasized stroke along the inside of the foot, starting from the arch and ending as you wrap around the heel before gently returning to the arch and starting again (see Fig. 5.13).

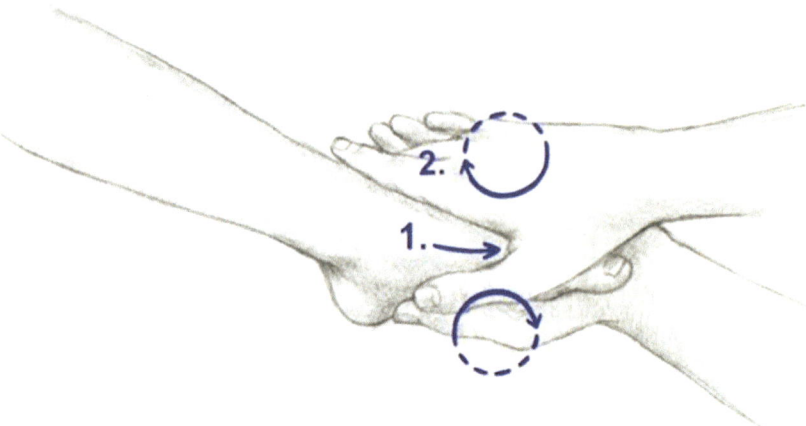

Fig. 5.12 Applying the oil to the foot and two-handed foot circles

Two-Handed Ankle Knuckle Circles
Release your hand from under the patient's foot, followed by the one above. One after the other, move both hands towards the back of the foot. Now slide the fingertips of both hands simultaneously down the outside and inside of the foot toward the ankle. Ease pressure lightly as you move upwards, but maintain skin contact. With an emphasized touch, circle the ankle knuckles moving from bottom to top. Once at the top, lighten the touch slightly. From there, gently return your hands to the starting position in a flowing motion. Repeat several times (see Fig. 5.14).

One-Handed Oil Application to the Foot
To end the foot embrocation, apply oil with one hand.

Return the hand nearest to the patient to near the Achilles tendon and lift the foot slightly. Leading with the fingertips, use the other hand, to apply light pressure from the base of the big toe over the sole of the foot toward the heel and beyond.

Repeat, but this time begin from the base of the little toe and then repeat once again starting from the base of the middle toe. After that, cover the foot and remove the support hand (see Fig. 5.15).

5.3.14 Figure Eight for the Foot

- *Effects*: releasing, warming, calming.
- *Indications*: tension, centralization, difficulty falling asleep, pre-active stage of dying.
- *Patient Position*: supine/sitting.

Fig. 5.13 Heel circle

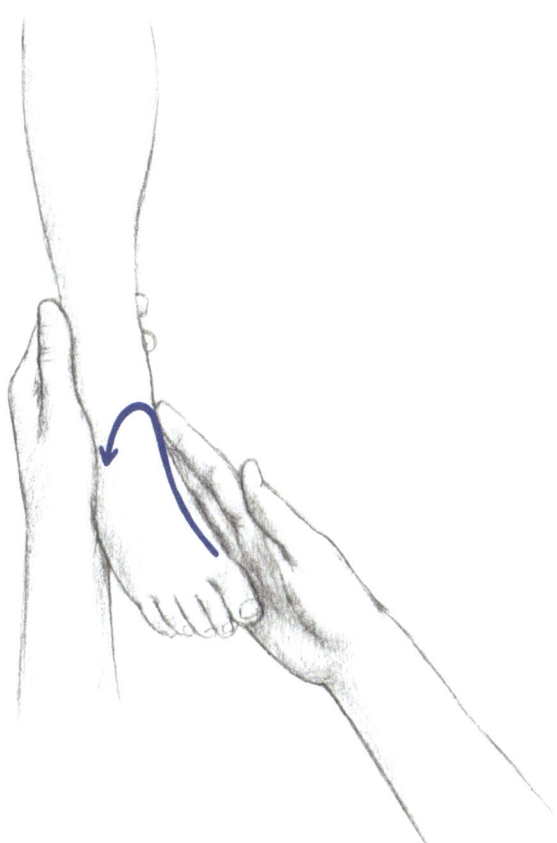

- *Practitioner Position*: to the side of the patient, next to the foot about to be treated.
- *Note*: can be used as an alternative for the multi-step foot embrocation (for example, when there is a lack of time).

Using the hand furthest from the patient, support their foot from the underside of the calf just above the Achilles tendon. To begin the figure eight, dip your other hand into the arch of their foot just below the base of their big toe. Stroke diagonally downward to the outside of the heel. Once there, circle the patient's heel with your fingers while keeping the heel of your hand in constant skin contact with the heel of their foot.

From the inside of their (foot) heel, lead with the heel of your hand, making an upward diagonal stroke to the ball of their foot. As your fingertips reach the area beneath their little toe, continue the stroke along the ball of the foot, returning to the original starting position. Repeat.

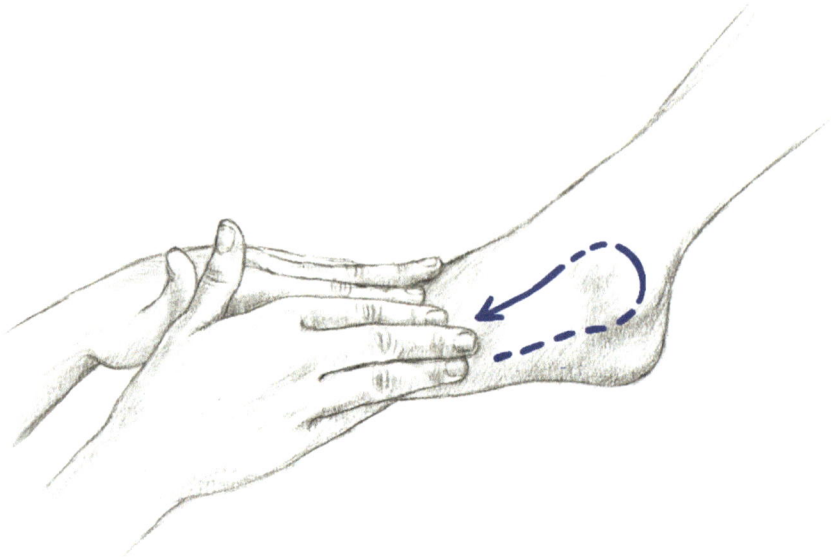

Fig. 5.14 Two-handed knuckle circling

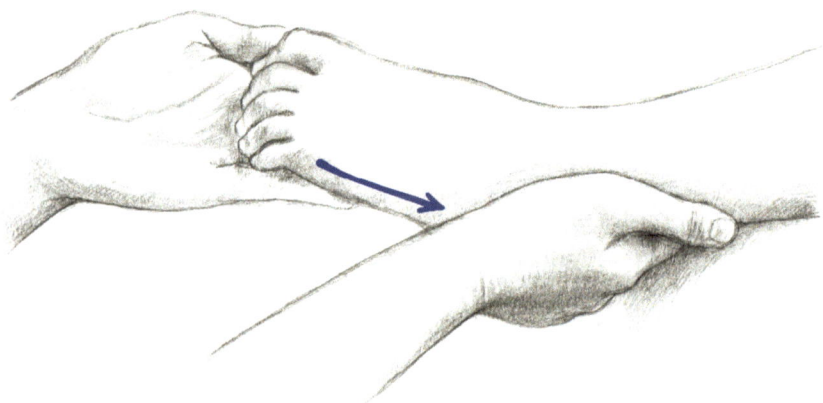

Fig. 5.15 One-handed oil application on the foot

5.3.15 Pentagram Embrocation

- *Effects*: invigorating, strengthening, clarifying.
- *Indications*: postoperative transit syndrome, depression, cardiac arrhythmias, after traumatic experiences, palliative situations, agitation/anxiety in the dying process.

- *Patient Position*: supine.
- *Practitioner Position*: stand facing the body area to be treated.
- *Note*: The patient's bed should be positioned so that you can approach from all sides. If this is not possible, remain on the accessible side of the bed and walk around the patient "in thought" while working.

In a pentagram embrocation, sometimes also called five-star embrocation, five points of the patient's periphery (head, hands, and feet) are rubbed with the chosen substance, one after another in a specific order. In this way, awareness is first directed to individual points and subsequently throughout the entire body.

Start with rubbing the forehead: using the index, middle and ring fingers of one hand perform three counterclockwise circles in the center of the forehead just above the nose.

Follow with seven counterclockwise circles, performed in the same way on the lower right leg above the ankle, and then wrap the right foot with a muslin cloth.

Next, do seven clockwise circles above the left wrist, and then wrap the hand in a muslin cloth.

Follow with seven counterclockwise circles on the right wrist, and then wrap the right hand with a muslin cloth, followed by seven clockwise circles on the left lower leg above the ankle followed by wrapping the foot.

Do a final three clockwise circles on the forehead.

To end the embrocation, place your right hand above the bed cover and lightly press on the patient's heart area for the duration of one breath, while gently placing your left hand on their forehead at the hairline. After the duration of one breath, slowly remove both of your hands from the patient.

5.4   Rhythmic Embrocation for Infants

One of the first sensory organs to develop in the womb is the sense of touch. Thus, the embryo begins to perceive the enveloped surrounding and boundary of the womb and amniotic fluid at an early stage. By building on these intrauterine experiences, an infant can be given a gentle start into life.

A special type of rhythmic embrocation is necessary for infants through which the newborn not only learns to feel itself and perceive its limitations, but also to smell and connect these experiences to each other.

5.4.1   Technique

Building upon the prenatal experiences of an infant does not require complex sequences or forms during a rhythmic embrocation. Rather, the focus is almost exclusively on using enveloping touches, which open slightly and close again, so that a certain warmth between the hands, and a breathing quality to the gestures are created. Due to this special quality of touch, rhythmic embrocations on infants are often referred to as *warming breaths* and not as embrocations at all. This approach is also due to the small body surface of infants [1].

Another special feature when working on infants is the sequence of treatments. In contrast to the treatment of other age groups, embrocations on infants are carried out from the periphery to the center. This too is based on embryonic development. Because of the small space and the fetal position of the unborn, the hands of the embryo grow from the periphery towards the heart, and the feet grow toward the navel [1].

Additionally, as a newborn's sense of smell is very pronounced, the substances and essential oils should only be dosed sparingly and usually diluted with a neutral oil. A more detailed description of the suitable dosages can be found in Chap. 6, Indications, listed according to individual indications.

5.4.2   Required Materials

The smaller the child or the younger the patient, the more they must be protected from cooling down. A heat lamp is therefore recommended. Furthermore, special attention should be paid to ensuring that the practitioners' hands are warm.

Materials Needed
- Support: couch, bed, or similar at working height.
- Blankets to cover areas of the body which are not being treated.
- Outer wrapping, use a cotton cloth or hand towel.
- Socks.
- Substance, essential oils, depending on the indication.
- Neutral vegetable oil, e.g., olive, almond, or sunflower oil, for diluting substances/finished preparations, as needed.
- Heat lamp, as needed.
- Hot water bottle to warm the hands of the practitioner, as needed.

5.4.3   Rhythmic Embrocation for Infants (Warming Breaths)

- *Effects*: calming, creates confidence/sense of security.
- *Indications*: fidgety/restless infants, jumpiness.
- *Patient Position*: supine.
- *Note*: This following application can also be done over clothing without using oil.

Each step described below can be done separately or can be performed sequentially in the order described.

Making Contact—Touching of the Head
To begin, make contact with the patient by positioning your arms to the left and right of the infant. Place your hands next to the infant's head with your palms facing

down, your thumb and index finger should have light skin contact with the patient. The infant's arms should be resting on top of yours. Now turn your palms inward toward the patient, gently embracing their head and slowly lift slightly from the bed. This creates a loving, enveloping gesture of affection. Hold this position for a short time and then release by slowly reversing each step.

Warming Breaths on the Foot
While the infant remains on their back, use your hands to gently enclose both feet from above and below, using your fingers to lightly support the ankles and lower legs. Use your upper hand to perform a circular motion in a clockwise direction, gently press your hands together on the back of the foot. As you move toward the toes, the touch should become gentler. Once finished, put socks on the infants' feet (see Fig. 5.16).

Warming Breaths on the Lower Legs
You can now proceed to the lower legs. Enclose both of the lower legs with your hands coming from the patients' outer sides. Your thumbs should rest gently in the direction of the knees. Slowly guide your thumbs toward each other so that the skin between them is lightly compressed. Afterwards, release by slightly opening the thumbs outwards without losing contact with the skin. This creates an upward opening gesture, a so-called breath gesture. Your movements should be very small, more a suggestion than a full execution.

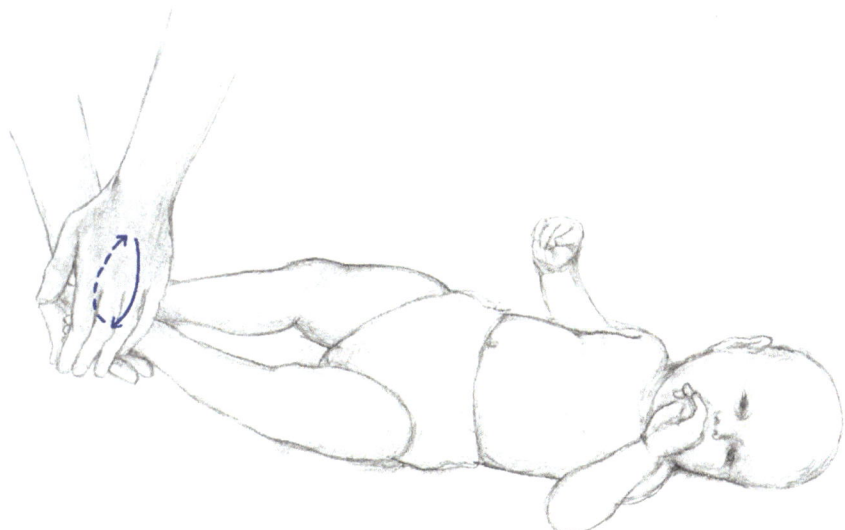

Fig. 5.16 Warming breaths on the foot

Warming Breaths on the Thigh

To move onto the thighs, place one hand after the other, on the outside of the thigh, your fingertips now resting on the infant's hip.

Perform the breath gestures on the thigh the same way as you did on the lower leg. To end, release both hands and cover the legs (see Fig. 5.17).

Warming Breaths on the Forearm

To continue, proceed to the arms beginning with the forearms. Rest your thumbs gently in the palms of the infants' hands. The infants' arms should begin in a position level with their chest. Using a gentle grip, bring their forearms in an arc outward toward the abdomen.

Warming Breath Circles on the Hand

Once the baby's hands reach their belly, enclose them with your hands. Use your fingers to gently make circle movements over the patient's fingers. Circle in an outward direction from the infant's body. Repeat several times. Slowly release touch by moving each hand, one after the other, to the outside of the patients' upper arms (see Fig. 5.18).

Warming Breaths on the Upper Arm

Position your hands so that your fingertips rest on the infant's shoulder joints and the heels of your hands are on their elbows. Slowly move both hands toward each other at the same time. Release at the same pace, without losing skin contact. The touch between the palms of your hands should be emphasized, with your fingers resting gently. Repeat several times. Release contact with both hands simultaneously.

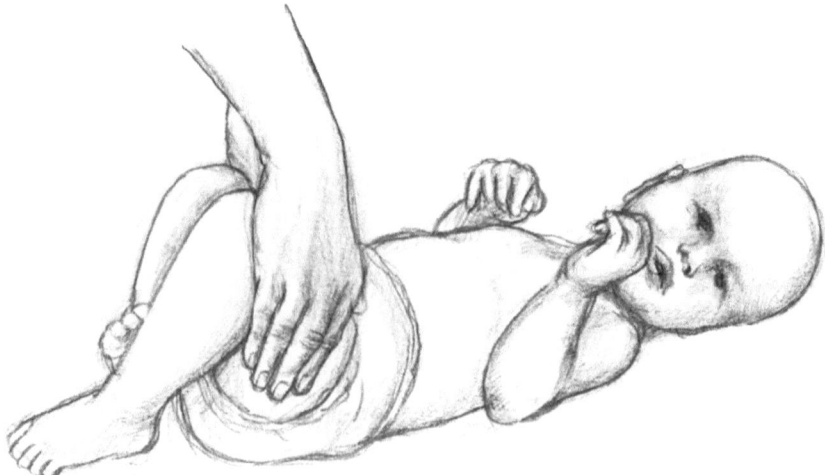

Fig. 5.17 Warming breaths on the thigh

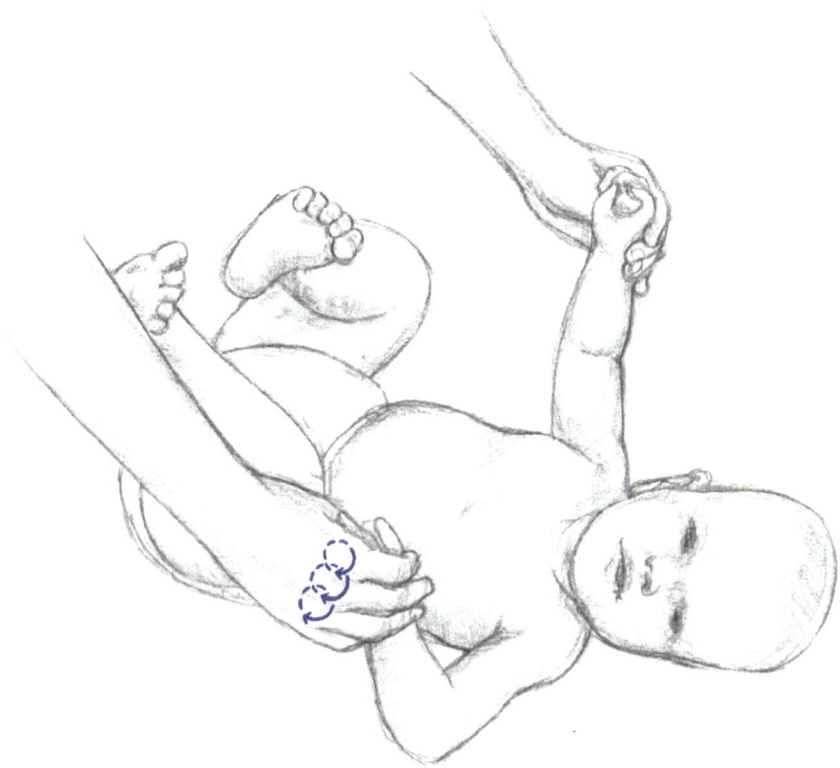

Fig. 5.18 Warmth circles on the hand

5.4.4 Two-Handed Back Circles for Infants

- *Effects*: calming, warming, deep breathing.
- *Indications*: restlessness, anxiety, respiratory disorders.
- *Patient Position*: prone position.
- *Note*: As a variation, the circling can also be done counterclockwise, this creates an inner balance and is particularly suitable for cardiac arrhythmias.

The infant should be positioned on their stomach on a surface allowing them to breathe comfortably. Place your warm (!) hands on the patients back so that the heels of your hands rest to the right and left of the infant's spine, with your fingers pointing outward, and gently wrapped around the patients' sides. Begin out-of-sync circles with both hands moving in a clockwise direction—but with the left beginning with a downward movement, while the right starts upward. The touch is emphasized (bound) as you move toward the outsides of the patient's body, and is eased (loosened) during the movement toward the spine. It is important to not touch or cross the spine during the treatment. Unlike back circles for other age groups, your hand should remain at one level and not move down the back.

Repeat several times. To end, use a slightly emphasized downward stroke toward the pelvis before releasing both hands simultaneously.

5.4.5 One-Handed Abdominal Circles for Infants

- *Effects*: antispasmodic, analgesic, mobilization of air in the intestine.
- *Indications*: constipation, meteorism, three-month colic, abdominal pain, hyperbilirubinemia.
- *Patient Position*: supine.
- *Note*: oils such as fennel, caraway, lemon balm, or yarrow oil are particularly suitable.

Depending on the size of the abdomen, use 1–4 fingers with light emphasis, to spiral clockwise around the belly button in increasingly larger circles. The area of the solar plexus should be left out entirely or touched only gently, otherwise it can lead to nausea and discomfort (see Fig. 5.19).

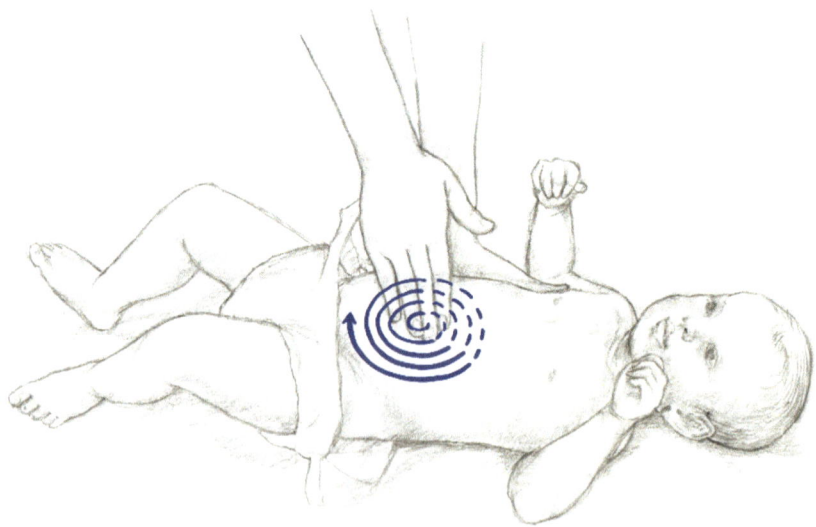

Fig. 5.19 One-handed abdominal circles

5.5   Compresses and Wrapped Compresses

Compresses are among the oldest forms of therapy; illustrations dating back as early as 1500 BC show hot Nile mud being used as a poultice [3]. They are quick to learn, easy to use and can be integrated well into everyday clinical practice. They are suitable for both mobile and immobile patients and are an ideal tool both for acute conditions and for chronic complaints, and in most cases do not require the continuous presence of the practitioner.

Both compresses and wrapped compress applications actually involve swathing a treated body area; however, the applications can be distinguished from each other by how the substance cloth (inner cloth) is used. In a *wrapped compress application, the entire treated area of the body is wrapped circularly with the substance cloth*, whereas, in a *compress application, the substance cloth is simply placed on top of the treated area* (see Fig. 5.20).

In both applications, an outer layer is wrapped around the area of the body treated. Depending on the substance being used, additional layers may be necessary, for example, a towel under the patient to protect the bed or a middle layer between the substance cloth and outer layer to protect wetness from seeping through.

Following either type of compress application, a post-treatment rest period of at least 15–20 min is recommended to support the healing process.

Compresses are particularly suitable for use in pediatrics because children can remain mobile with them and bed rest is not necessarily indicated.

The effects of compresses can be explained by various factors. On the one hand, by the substances used themselves, which act through their ingredients and/or through their ability to store heat/cold and slowly release it to the body. On the other hand, the targeted use of heat or cold creates a physical effect that influences blood circulation. Additionally, the (usually) pleasant scent emanating from the compress and the feeling of security it gives, can make an essential contribution to the healing process.

Fig. 5.20 Oil compress, warm pack

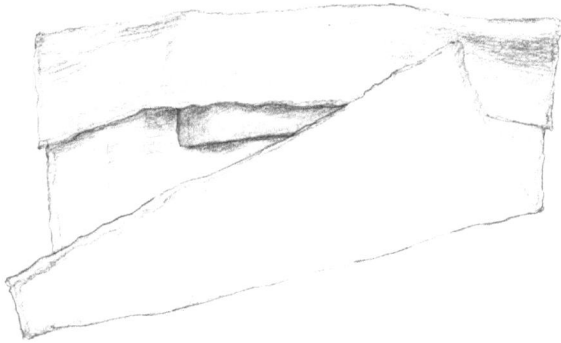

5.5.1 Oil Compresses

- *Effects*: depending on substance used (see substance chapter).
- *Indications*: depending on substance used (see substance chapter).
- *Contraindications*: unclear abdomen, defective skin, inflammatory processes, fever.
- *Patient Position*: depending on the indication.
- *Duration*: min. 20 min, 30 min post rest.
- *Note*: since there is no evaporative cooling, an oil compress can also be applied overnight.
- *Attention*: Oil heats up very quickly, therefore a temperature check before use is absolutely necessary!

Material Needed
- Substance cloth, made of cotton (smaller than the warm pack).
- Outer wrap (large cotton cloth/towel/scarf)—or.
- in the case of infants, a onesie can be used instead,
- Substance according to the indication (your mix of essential oils and neutral vegetable oil or a ready-to-use preparation).
- Warm pack (a wool cloth wrapped inside a cotton cloth so that the fibers won't irritate the skin).
- Small bowl and spoon, if necessary.
- Re-sealable bag/plastic bag.
- 1–2 hot-water bottles
- Adhesive tape.

Preparation
If you are using your own mixture of an essential oil and a neutral vegetable oil, place the substance cloth in the freezer bag first, drizzle with the oil mixture (preferably with pipette) and spread; the cloth should be well wetted, but not dripping. If you are using a ready-made preparation, drizzle the substance cloth with the selected oil in a random pattern which resembles a starry night sky and place it in a re-sealable bag (see Fig. 5.21).

Fill both hot-water bottles with 60–70 °C hot water (mix 2/3 boiling hot water with 1/3 cold water) and put both the warm pack and the substance cloth (still in the re-sealable bag) between them for 5–10 min.

The re-sealable bag protects the hot-water bottles from the essential oils and can also be used for storing the substance cloth post-treatment so it can be used more than once. The outer wrap can also be placed around the hot water bottles, so that it is also nicely warmed through (see Fig. 5.22).

Instructions for Implementation
Once the substance cloth and warm pack have been thoroughly warmed and are ready for use, place the outer wrap crosswise under the patient so that it protrudes

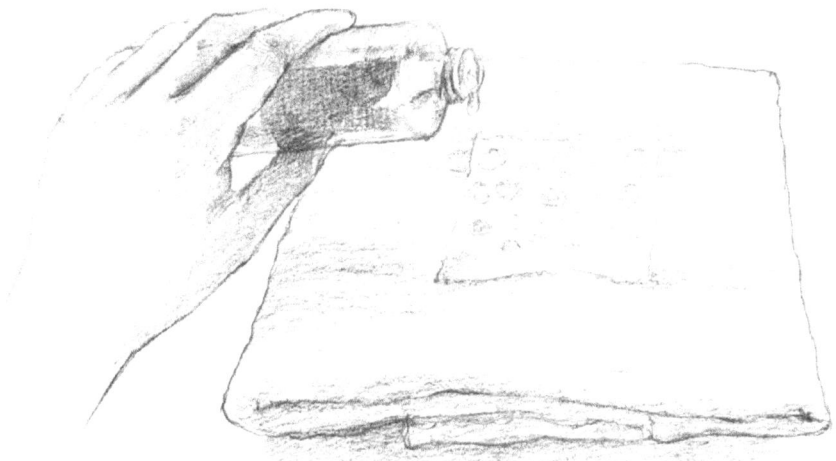

Fig. 5.21 Oil compress, drizzling ready-to-use preparation on substance cloth

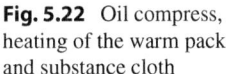

Fig. 5.22 Oil compress, heating of the warm pack and substance cloth

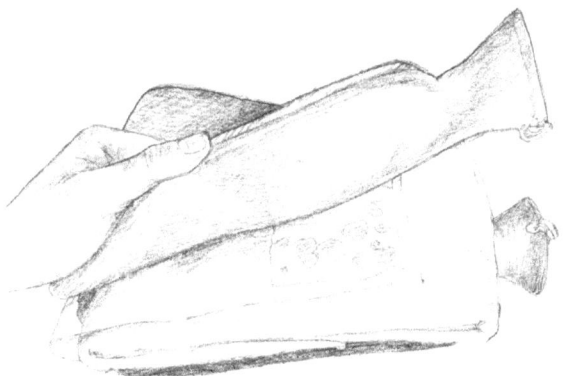

about the same length on both sides. Remove the substance cloth from the freezer bag and place directly on the area to be treated. Place the warm pack on top and swath in place using the outer wrap. You can use adhesive tape to fix everything in place (see Fig. 5.23).

For infants, the outer wrap can be replaced by a onesie. The application should be allowed to take effect for at least 20 min. Since there is no evaporative cooling, it can also be applied over a longer period, for example, overnight.

Following Treatment
Place the substance cloth back in the freezer bag after use, this helps retain the essential oils and the cloth can be used for 3–5 days without reapplying oil. If the scent has evaporated, a renewed light sprinkling with oil is sufficient.

Fig. 5.23 Oil compress, application on the patient

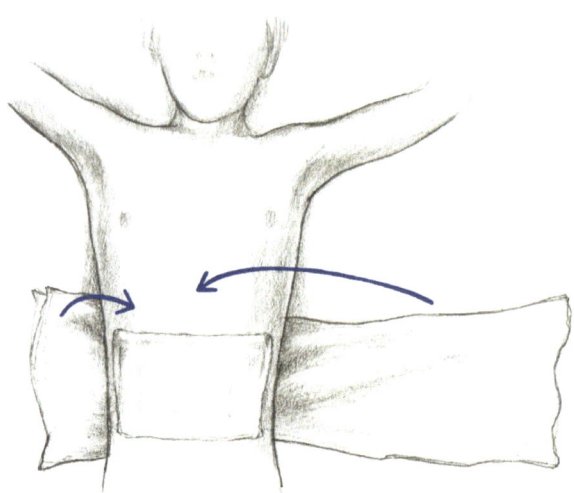

5.5.2 Warm/Hot (Moist) Compresses and Wrapped Compresses

- *Age Suitability*: warm wrapped compresses can be applied in infancy, but hot compresses are not suitable for children under the age of 6 years!
- *Effects*: stimulates blood circulation, metabolism, relaxing, antispasmodic.
- *Indications*: cough, bronchitis, constipation, flatulence, three-month colic.
- *Contraindications*: unclear abdomen, defective skin, inflammatory processes, fever, thrombocytopenia.
- *Patient Position*: supine.
- *Duration*: max. 10 min, 30 min post-treatment rest.
- *Note*: the younger the patient, the lower the temperature of application.
- *Attention*: The temperature must be checked before applying, otherwise there is a risk of scalding.

Materials Needed
- Substance cloth, made of cotton.
- Protective middle layer, made of cotton (to prevent seepage and reduce evaporative cooling).
- Outer wrap (large cotton cloth/towel/scarf).
- Wringing cloth (tea towel).
- Tea substance according to the indication (e.g., chamomile, lemon balm, yarrow).
- 1 liter 40 °C warm water (warm application)/1 liter 60 °C warm water (hot application)
- Large bowl.
- 1–2 hot-water bottles
- Adhesive Tape.

Preparation

Fold the substance cloth inward toward the center from all sides and place in the middle of the out-stretched tea towel cloth (see wringing cloth). Roll together so that the folded substance cloth is located *only* in the center of the tea towel. Use the hot water/tea to either douse the center area enveloping the substance cloth or to soak that section in a bowl. The ends of the tea towel should remain dry so as not to burn yourself. Holding the dry ends of the tea towel, twist to wring out the inner cloth (Fig. 5.24). The more the substance cloth is wrung out, the longer the heat will be retained and the better it will be tolerated by the patient.

Instructions for Implementation

Depending on which area of the body is to be treated, place the outer wrap at the chest/abdominal level of the patient's bed, and fold it over once at the middle. Place the protective middle layer on top. You can now use hot-water bottles to preheat the bed, to increase patient comfort.

Once the hot-water bottles have been removed and the patient has lain down, remove the substance cloth from the wringing towel. Check the temperature by dabbing the substance cloth on the inside of your forearm/wrist. If the temperature is comfortable, dab the body region of the patient that is to be treated so that they can adjust to the stimulus before quickly applying the substance cloth.

The substance cloth itself can either be wrapped around the areas to be treated or simply placed on top. Wrapping the substance cloth requires practice and is not suitable for children under the age of three.

Regardless of how the substance cloth is applied, cover it entirely with the protective middle layer and wrap tightly with the outer cloth, so no air can enter and cause evaporative cooling. For a better hold, the outer layer can be fixed with adhesive tape. Do not fix with pins because of the risk of injury.

The duration of application depends on the patient, but should not exceed 10 min to avoid cooling. During the application, the patient should be kept warm and well covered.

Fig. 5.24 Wringing out the substance cloth using a wringing cloth

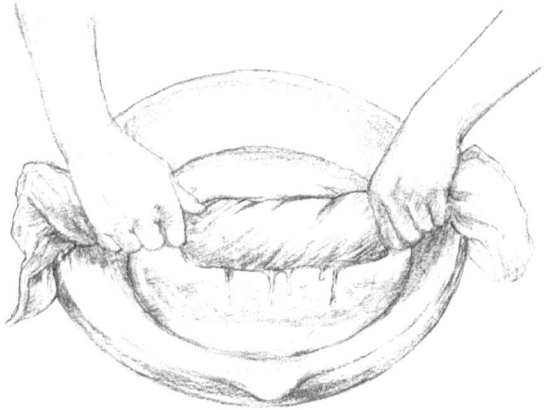

Following Treatment
Dry the treated body region well. A post-treatment rest of approx. 30 min is recommended.

5.5.3   Mustard Flour Compress

- *Age Suitability*: from 6 years onward.
- *Effects*: increases blood circulation, activates metabolic processes in the treated area, deepens the respiratory system, thereby increasing oxygen saturation in the blood, dissolves secretions.
- *Indications*: pneumonia,—prophylaxis, bronchitis, cold, painful joints, chronic. Spinal diseases, muscle tension.
- *Contraindications*: sensitive skin, open wounds, acute inflammation/sensitivity disorder in the area of application.
- *Patient Position*: sitting/supine.
- *Duration*: max. 10 min, 30 min post rest.
- *Note*: May also be used in cases of mild fever to help the body dissipate heat.
- *Caution*: Excessive duration of application may result in burns with blistering. A patient should not be left alone during the application!

Materials Needed
- Substance packet, use a cotton cloth with a paper towel inlay.
- Protective middle layer, made of cotton (to prevent seepage and reduce evaporative cooling).
- Outer wrap (large cotton cloth/towel/scarf).
- Wringing cloth (tea towel).
- Substance, 1–2, max. 3 tbsp black mustard flour.
- 30–40 °C warm water
- Large bowl.
- Petroleum jelly (to protect nipples in chest applications).
- 2 cotton pads (to protect nipples in chest applications)
- Thermos flask, if necessary.
- Nourishing oil.
- Clock.
- Hot-water bottle, if needed.

Preparation
Spread the mustard flour thinly and evenly on half of the paper towel, leaving the edges free. Fold the uncovered half of the paper towel over and fold all the edges inward so that no mustard flour can escape. Place in the middle of the cotton cloth, and fold sides inward to form a small packet (Fig. 5.25).

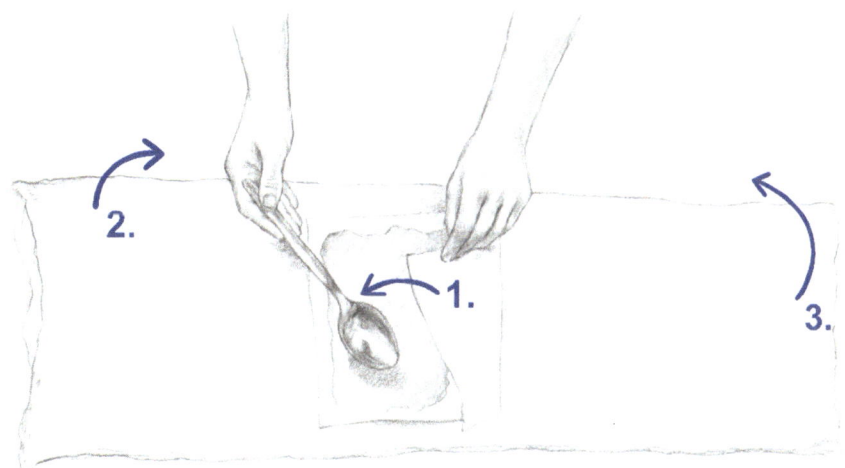

Fig. 5.25 Preparing the mustard compress

Place the substance packet in the middle of the outstretched tea towel cloth (wringing cloth). Roll together so that the folded inner cloth is located *only* in the center of the tea towel. Place in a bowl with 30–40 °C warm water, turning over several times. Be sure to keep the ends of the tea towel dry so that you will have a place to hold onto as you wring it out. To prevent the packet from cooling, keep it soaking in the bowl and remove only directly before application—while already beside the patient.

Instructions for Implementation

First, coat the patients' nipples with petroleum jelly and cover each with a cotton pad to protect them from the irritating effects of the mustard flour (for chest applications).

Explain to the patient that once the compress is applied they will quickly notice a tingling and then a burning sensation. These are desired effects but should be constantly monitored.

Wring out and then remove the substance cloth coated in mustard from the wringing cloth. Place the packet on the patient's chest or on the affected joint. Cover with the protective middle layer and wrap with the outer cloth.

After 1–2 min, check the skin. If there is even a slight redness, the compress should be removed immediately, otherwise burns may occur. If the skin still shows no reaction and the patient is tolerating it well, the compress may remain in place. After another 1–2 min, check the skin again. If no skin reaction can be detected, and the patient continues to tolerate the application, the compress can be left in place for another 10 min.

If the patient has cold feet, a hot water bottle with 60 °C water (2/3 boiling hot water mixed with 1/3 cold water) can be placed near the feet during the application and the post-treatment rest.

Following Treatment
After removing the compress, rub the application area with a nourishing oil and re-wrap the area with the towel for a post-treatment rest of 30 min.

5.5.4 Horseradish Compress

- *Age Suitability*: from 8 years onward.
- *Effects*: secretion release, warming, increases blood circulation.
- *Indications*: sinusitis, rhinitis, headache.
- *Contraindications*: sensitive skin, open wounds, acute inflammation/sensitivity disorder in the area of application.
- *Patient Position*: sitting/supine/side/belly position.
- *Duration*: 1–5 min, 30 min post-treatment rest.
- *Frequency*: 1x daily.
- *Note*: The patient should not be left alone during treatment due to the irritating effects of the substance. In case of strong heat development, burning and strong reddening of the skin, the compress should be removed immediately!
- *Caution*: application that is applied too long may cause burns and damage to the nerve cells in the skin.

Materials Needed
- Substance cloth (thin cotton cloth about 15 × 15 cm/paper tissue).
- Outer wrap (medium sized cotton cloth or scarf).
- Substance, 1 tsp. freshly grated horseradish root.
- Nourishing oil.

Preparation
Spread the freshly grated horseradish over the center of the substance cloth, leaving the edges free. Fold the uncovered half of the paper towel over and fold all the edges inward so that no horseradish can escape, forming a small packet.

Instructions for Implementation
Explain to the patient that once the compress is applied they will quickly notice a tingling and then a burning sensation. These are desired effects but should be constantly monitored.

Place the substance packet on the neck area between the sixth and seventh cervical vertebrae, with the single-layered side facing the skin. The packet should be held in place by you or the patient themself.

After 1–2 min, check the skin. If there is even a slight redness, the compress should be removed immediately, otherwise burns may occur. If the skin still shows no reaction and the patient is tolerating it well, the compress may remain in place. After another 1–2 min check the skin again. If no skin reaction can be detected, and the patient continues to tolerate the application, the compress can be left in place for a maximum of 5 min.

Following Treatment
After removing the compress, rub the application area with a nourishing oil and wrap the area with the outer cloth and leave in place for a post-treatment rest of 30 min.

5.5.5   Ginger Compress and Wrapped Ginger Compress for Chest

- *Age Suitability*: from 2 years onward.
- *Effects*: expectorant, warming, analgesic, stimulation of diuresis.
- *Indications*: bronchitis, pneumonia, asthma, arthritis, kidney diseases, muscle tension, back pain, cold states, restlessness.
- *Contraindications*: fever, hypertension, sensitive skin, acute inflammation/sensitivity disorder in the area of application.
- *Patient Position*: supine/side/belly position.
- *Duration*: 20–40 min, post-treatment rest for 30 min.
- *Frequency*: 1× daily (preferably in the morning).
- *Note*: the patient should not be left alone during treatment due to the irritating effects of the substance. If strong heat develops, with burning and strong reddening of the skin, remove the compress and reduce the amount of substance used next time!
- *Attention*: any redness from the previous treatment should have completely subsided before the next application!

Materials Needed
- Substance cloth, made of cotton.
- Protective middle layer, made of cotton (to prevent seepage and reduce evaporative cooling).
- Towel or waterproof pad to protect the bed (in wrapped chest applications).
- Outer wrap (large cotton cloth/towel/scarf).
- Wringing cloth (tea towel).
- Substance, ginger powder (from 2 years ½ tsp., from 6 years 1 tsp., from 12 years 1 tbsp.)
- 75 °C hot water
- Small bowl.
- Vaseline (to protect nipples in chest wrap applications).
- Two cotton pads (to protect nipples in chest wrap applications)
- Nourishing oil.

Preparation

In a small bowl, mix the ginger powder with 300–400 ml of hot water and leave to infuse. After 3–5 min, dip the substance cloth into the bowl and soak it. If a weaker stimulus is required, the substance cloth can be wrapped in the wringing cloth before soaking.

Instructions for Implementation

Compress

Wring out the substance cloth using the tea towel as a wringing cloth. Apply to the area in pain or kidney region (depending on the indication). The application temperature should be as hot as can be tolerated. Cover with the towel (middle layer). Without wrinkles, wrap the area snugly with the outer layer. Cover the patient with a blanket to prevent evaporative cooling.

Wrapped Compress for the Chest

First, place a large towel under the patient's back to protect the bed. At the patient's chest level on top, place the outer wrap, followed by the protective middle layer. The patient lies on top of all 3 layers, with their upper body exposed. Coat the patient's nipples with Vaseline and cover each with a cotton pad to protect them from the irritating effects of the ginger. Using the wringing cloth, wring out the substance cloth. The application temperature should be warm but not hot. Place the substance cloth on the chest so that it wraps around to the patient's back without wrinkling and does not cover the spine. Cover the compress entirely with the middle towel and wrap tightly with the outer layer so that no evaporative cooling can occur. Finally, cover the patient with a blanket.

Following Treatment

After 20–40 min, remove the compress and rub the application area with a nourishing or pain-relieving oil. Wrap the area again with the outer layer for a post-treatment rest of 30 min.

5.5.6 Cool (Moist) Wrapped Compresses

- *Age*: pulse wraps from 1 month of age; calf wraps from 6 months of age.
- *Effects*: cooling.
- *Indications*: Fever.
- *Patient Position*: sitting/supine.
- *Duration*: 1530 min, 15–30 min post rest.
- *Note*: A maximum temperature drop of 0.5–1 °C is aimed for, the temperature continues to drop during the resting phase.
- *Caution*: circulatory problems and risk of hypothermia if used too long or if application is too cold.

Cool wrapped compresses are an ideal way to gently reduce fever, especially in children. It is important that they are applied only at peak of the fever and when the extremities are warm. As a fever rises, body heat is centralized and the extremities feel cold, meaning no heat release is possible through the periphery during this phase.

Since infants and young children have a larger body surface area in relation to their body weight than adults, there is a risk that the body temperature will drop too quickly, which can put a strain on the circulation system. Therefore, patients should not be left alone during a cool wrapped compress application and their temperature should be monitored. The application temperature should not be too cold. The water temperature should be about 2–3 °C below body temperature, and for infants and toddlers, only 1–2 °C (the younger the child, the smaller the temperature difference there should be!).

However, the point to which the fever must be lowered depends on the patient's condition and the underlying disease, and is therefore subject to doctors' orders.

Cool (Moist) Wrapped Compress for the Calf
Materials Needed
- 2 substance cloths made of cotton
- 2–3 terry towels
- Bath thermometer.
- Bowl filled with cool water, adjusted according to the patient's body temperature (see above).
- Clinical thermometer (to check the patient's temperature before and after use).

Instructions for Implementation
After taking the patient's temperature, place a towel under the patient's calves to protect the bed. Then dip the substance cloths into the bowl filled with water (for temperature, see above) until they are completely soaked. Wring out well. Snugly wrap each calf with one of the substance cloths, without wrinkling. If necessary, wrap an additional terry towel around the calves or place loosely over both legs.

Do not cover the lower legs with anything else, so as not to disturb the cooling effect of the compresses. However, cover the patient's torso with a blanket so that they do not freeze.

Remove the compresses as soon as they have warmed (after about 5–10 min.), and soak again in the cool water, and repeat the application. This procedure can be repeated three to a maximum of four times before measuring the patient's body temperature once again.

Following the Treatment
The patient should then rest for another 15–30 min.

Cool (Moist) Wrapped Compress for the Wrist
Materials Needed
- 2 substance cloths (handkerchiefs work well)
- 2 wrist warmers/socks/small cloths

- Bath thermometer.
- Small bowl with cool water (adjusted to patient's body temperature).
- Clinical thermometer (to check the patient's temperature before and after use).
- Adhesive tape.

Instructions for Implementation
Dip the substance cloths into the water (for temperature see above). Wring out well. Now wrap them around the wrists of the patient. To fix them, use a wrist band, a sock pulled over the hand, or wrap with a small cloth and fix with adhesive tape.

Remove the compresses as soon as they have warmed (after about 5–10 min.), and soak again in the cool water, and repeat the application. This procedure can be repeated three to a maximum of four times before measuring the patient's body temperature once again.

Following the Treatment
The patient should then rest for a further 10–20 min.

5.5.7 Farmers Cheese (Quark) Compresses/ Wrapped Compresses

- *Age Suitability*: from 1 month of age.
- *Effects*: antispasmodic and expectorant, decongestant, respiratory deepening, cooling.
- *Indications*: Sore throat, cough, bronchitis, inflammations, bruise, sprain, sunburn, insect bites, itching, bruises.
- *Contraindications*: neurodermatitis, cow's milk allergy.
- *Patient Position*: supine/sitting.
- *Duration*: 2–3 h/overnight if necessary, 15–30 min post-treatment rest.
- *Note*: the cheese should not come into direct contact with the skin.
- *Caution*: If the cheese is too cold, there is a risk of hypothermia. For a cool application (e.g., neck compress) the cheese should be room temperature. For large-area torso applications (e.g., chest compress), it should be warmed to body temperature (see below).

Materials Needed
- Substance packet, use a cotton cloth a bit larger than the area to be treated, with a paper towel inlay.
- Protective middle layer, made of cotton (to prevent seepage and reduce evaporative cooling).
- Towel or waterproof pad to protect for the bed.
- Outer wrap (cotton cloth/towel/scarf size depending on area to be treated).
- Substance 50–100 g farmers cheese (room temperature!)
- Wooden spatula/knife.
- Hot-water bottle (for wrapped chest compress).
- Nourishing cream/oil, if necessary.

Preparation

Use a spatula to spread the cheese about ½–1 cm thick on the paper towel matching the area to be treated. The edges should be left free and folded inward toward the center to form a small packet. The cheese should not have direct contact with the skin, as patients perceive this as unpleasant.

Instructions for Implementation
Wrapped Compress for the Neck.

The substance packet should be sized to cover the front and side part of the neck, but leave the spine free. Place on the neck with the single-layered side on the skin and wrap with the outer cloth. If necessary, a scarf can be used.

Chest Compress (Warm)

For a chest application, the cheese should be heated to about 36–37 °C (body temperature) using a water bath, stirring constantly. The substance packet should be large enough to reach from the patient's armpit to their lower ribcage. To prevent it from cooling down before application, it can be kept warm with a hot-water bottle.

As an alternative to heating in a water bath, you can use hot-water bottles. To do this, place the prepared substance packet between two hot-water bottles with a temperature of approx. 60 °C, for 20 min. The hot-water bottles should not be hotter than 60 °C, otherwise the protein will coagulate and the whey will evaporate.

First, place a large towel under the patient's back to protect the bed. At the patient's chest level, place the outer wrap on top, followed by the protective middle layer. The patient lies on top of all 3 layers, with their upper body exposed, placed directly on top of it at chest level.

Place the substance packet on the patient's chest and cover with the protective middle layer, wrap the outer cloth around the chest and cover the patient with a blanket.

Compress (Cool)

Place the cool substance packet directly on the affected area (e.g., bruises or insect bites) with the single-layer side facing the skin. This is often sufficient on its own, but, if necessary, you can wrap it with an outer cloth.

All types of quark compresses can be applied for either 2–3 h, or even overnight, if necessary, but should be removed earlier if the patient is uncomfortable or cold, or if the cheese has dried out.

In acute situations, the compress should be applied 1–maximum 2 times a day.

Following Treatment

If the skin in the treated area is dry, rub the area with a nourishing cream or oil. The patient should rest for another 15–30 min.

5.5.8 Lemon Slice Compress

- *Age Suitability*: from 2 years of age.
- *Effects*: decongestant, expectorant, antipyretic, anti-inflammatory.
- *Indications for Neck Compress*: sore throat, pharyngitis, tonsillitis.

- *Indications for Foot Sole Compress*: fever, headache.
- *Patient Position*: sitting/lying.
- *Duration*: neck compress: 30 min; foot sole compress: 15 min, 15–30 min post-treatment rest.
- *Note*: Lemon can be irritating to the skin. The compress should be removed immediately in case of itching or burning and the skin should be cleaned with lukewarm water.
- *Caution*: Do not use this application on sensitive skin.

Materials Needed
- Substance packet, use a cotton cloth with a paper towel inlay.
- Outer wrap, use a cotton cloth or scarf.
- Gauze bandage (for foot sole support).
- Substance, 1 untreated lemon.
- Board and knife.
- Fever thermometer, if needed.

Preparation
Wash the lemon, cut it into thin slices, and place next to each other in the center of the substance packet. Fold inward from all sides and press so that some juice is squeezed out with the heel of your hand. The packet size should correspond to the area of the patient to be treated.

Instructions for Implementation
Neck Compress
The substance packet should be sized to cover the front and side part of the neck, but leave the spine free. Place on the neck with the single-layered side to the skin and wrap with the outer cloth. If necessary, a scarf can be used.

After 30 min, remove the compress and dry the neck. Depending on the patient's needs, a scarf can be put back on to keep the neck warm.

Compress for the Foot Sole
Place a substance packet on each foot sole and wrap in place with a gauze bandage. Put socks on the patients' feet.

After 15 min, remove the compresses and replace the socks.

Following Treatment
The patient should then rest for another 15–30 min.

5.5.9   Onion Bags for the Ear

- *Age*: from 1 year of age.
- *Effects*: analgesic, anti-inflammatory, decongestant, expectorant.

- *Indications*: earache, otitis media.
- *Contraindications*: defective skin in the area of application.
- *Patient Position*: sitting/lying.
- *Duration*: 30–60 min, 30–60 min post-treatment rest.
- *Note*: If well tolerated, the onion bags can be left on for up to 2 h and can be used up to twice a day if needed.

Materials Needed
- Substance cloth, a cloth handkerchief works well.
- Outer wrap, use a headband/cap/ scarf.
- Substance, 1 onion diced.
- String/adhesive tape, if needed.
- Freezer bag.
- Hot-water bottle filled with approx. 60–70 °C warm water (mix 2/3 boiling hot water with 1/3 cold water).

Preparation
Spread the finely diced onion on the substance cloth. Fold the edges inward to form a small packet and place in a freezer bag. Warm to the patient's body temperature using the hot water bottle. If necessary, the bag can be closed with a string or adhesive tape so that no pieces of onion can fall out.

Instructions for Implementation
The warmed packet is now removed from the freezer bag and placed on the painful ear and around the auricle and secured with a headband or something similar.

The compress should remain on the ear for at least 30–60 min, but if well-tolerated, can also be applied for up to 2 h.

Following Treatment
Afterwards, carefully clean the ear with lukewarm water to reduce the odor. A rest period of 30–60 min is recommended.

5.5.10 Arnica Cap

- *Age Suitability*: from 3 years of age.
- *Effects*: restorative, regulating, ordering of sensory perception.
- *Indications*: headache.
- *Contraindications*: arnica intolerance.
- *Patient Position*: supine.
- *Duration*: 30–45 min, 30–60 min post-treatment rest.
- *Note*: If the patient's hair is still wet afterwards, it should be dried.

Material
- Substance cloth, use a small wash cloth.
- Outer wrap, use a large towel/cotton cloth.
- Substance, 1 tbsp arnica essence.
- 250 ml lukewarm water
- Bowl.

Preparation
Mix one tablespoon of arnica essence with about 250 ml of lukewarm water. The temperature of the water can be adapted to the patient's wishes. Fold the substance cloth to a size corresponding to the size of the patient's forehead and soak in the arnica mixture and then wring out.

Instructions for Implementation
The patient should lie comfortably on their back. Fold the outer wrap into a triangle and place under the patient's head, with the top corner protruding out and pointing toward the top end of the bed. The other two corners should be protruding out from under the head, parallel to the patients' shoulders.

Place the substance cloth on the patient's forehead. Fold the top corner of the outer wrapping cloth down onto the patient's forehead, and fold each lateral corner on top, the hair should be covered and the wrap should almost look like a hood. If necessary, you can fix the ends in place with adhesive tape, or alternatively, a cap can be put over it. The eyes can be lightly covered as long as the patient feels comfortable (Fig. 5.26).

Following Treatment
After 15–20 min, remove the substance cloth. The outer wrapping cloth may remain in place for the post-treatment rest of approx. 15–30 min.

5.5.11 Rosemary Socks

- *Age Suitability*: premature infants from 28 weeks of gestation.
- *Effects*: invigorating, strengthening, vitalizing.
- *Indications*: primary apneas, respiratory distress syndrome, bradycardia tendency, sleepiness, fatigue, drowsiness.
- *Patient Position*: supine/lateral/prone position.
- *Duration*: 2 h, 30 min post-treatment rest.

Materials Needed
- 2 Substance cloths—approximately 5 × 5 cm
- 2 Outer wraps, cloths approximately 10 × 10 cm
- Substance, Rosemary ointment 1%.
- Adhesive tape.
- Wooden spatula.
- Wool socks.

Fig. 5.26 Arnica Cap

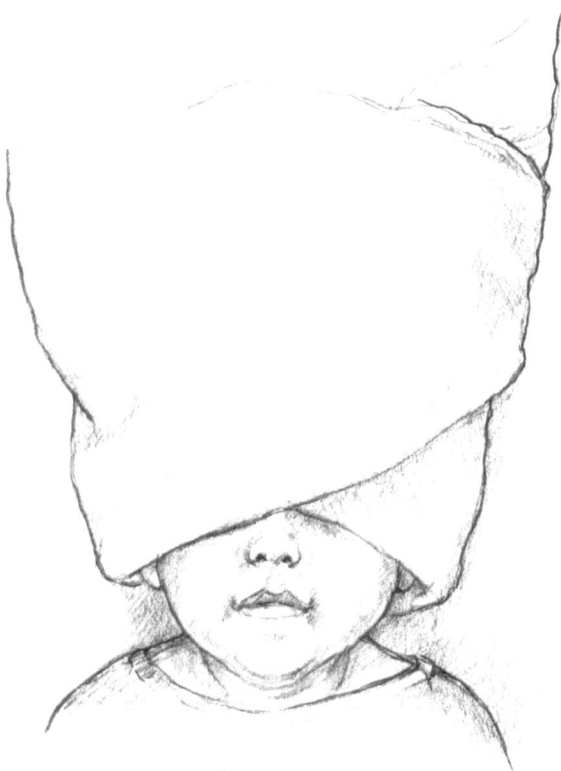

Preparation
Using a spatula, prepare the two substance cloths by spreading rosemary ointment about 1–2 mm thick, so that the substance looks almost like a shiny mirror.

Instructions for Implementation
Apply the substance cloth directly to the sole of each foot, wrap with the outer cloth and fix with adhesive tape, if necessary. Put on wool socks on the patient to keep their feet warm.

Following Treatment
After 2 h, remove the compresses and then put the wool socks back on. A post-treatment rest of 30 min is recommended.

5.6   Therapeutic Washes and Baths

Washes and baths can be used for more than removing dirt. They can combine cleaning and care, and can have a therapeutic effect with the addition of a substance. Depending on the temperature and the substance used, washes and baths can have either a calming or stimulating effect [5, 4].

Even before birth, we are surrounded by amniotic fluid and thus closely connected with the element of water. Through its buoyant forces, water triggers a feeling of lightness and a sense of security in us.

Due to the many different types of washes and baths, even seriously ill patients with limited mobility can benefit from the effects of water and the various substances.

Substances can be teas made from medicinal plants, bath milk, or oils (essential, as well as fatty oils). However, oils should never be added directly to water, because the fat molecules cannot combine with the water. Therefore, an emulsion of oil and cream/coffee cream should be used (1 tablespoon (tbsp) of oil to 1–2 tbsp of cream, or alternatively, milk). In case of milk allergy, vegetable cream (e.g., soy cream) or honey can be used instead, (1–2 tbsp honey to 1 tbsp oil).

The effects of the substances can be found in the Chap. 7, Substances.

5.6.1   Therapeutic Whole-Body Wash

- *Effects*: invigorating, stimulates blood circulation/soothing, enveloping.
- *Indications*: cleaning, constant fatigue/restlessness.
- *Patient Position*: supine/side position/seated.
- *Duration*: 10–15 min.
- *Note*: After washing individual body parts, they should be dried immediately and then covered/wrapped warmly.

Therapeutic washes are ideal for providing direct communication with patients who experience quantitative disorders of consciousness or loss of sensory stimuli. However, patients who have none of these limitations can also benefit from a therapeutic wash.

Before a therapeutic wash begins, you must decide upon the desired effect. This will determine how the wash is performed and which substance is used. A therapeutic wash can be used to either stimulate or calm.

Always begin with the head, specifically with the forehead of the patient. In order to achieve the greatest possible effect, each touch should be performed calmly, with the entire palm of the hand and using constant pressure.

After washing individual body parts, they should be dried immediately and then wrapped to prevent cooling as you continue with the wash.

The mouth and the intimate areas, are not included in the therapeutic washing, they should be cleaned beforehand or afterwards.

Materials Needed
- Washing bowl.
- Bath thermometer.
- Substance.
- Washcloth.

- Towels.
- Blanket.

Stimulating Wash

A stimulating wash is performed with cool water (35–38 °C, approximately the patient's body temperature) washing from the patient's periphery to their center. Use stroking movements in the opposite direction of hair growth to increase awareness and clarity. This can help create a sense of self as separate from the outside world.

As already mentioned, start with the patient's forehead, followed by their right hand, forearm, upper arm and armpit. Continue with the left hand, forearm, upper arm, and armpit. Next, wash the chest and abdomen. Wash the back from top to bottom along the spine.

Once the entire upper body has been washed, you can move onto the lower body, beginning with the patient's right-hand side, wash in the following sequence: foot, lower leg, knee, and finally thigh, before moving on to their left side.

Soothing Wash

For a soothing wash, use water about 8–10 °C above the patient's body temperature. This type of therapeutic wash begins at the patient's center and moves outward to their periphery. Use circular movements in the direction of hair growth to give the patient a calming feeling of being enveloped. This type of washing has a warming character.

Again, start with the patient's head, followed by their chest and abdomen, and then back. Continue with the left upper arm, forearm and hand and then do the same on their right side. After the arms, start with the left leg and then the right leg in the order of thigh, knee, lower leg, and foot.

5.6.2   Tinkling Wash

- *Effects*: calming, clarifying, releasing, giving security/hope.
- *Indications*: very weak, immobile patients, palliative, agitation, anxiety.
- *Patient Position*: supine/sitting.
- *Duration*: according to the needs of the patient.
- *Note*: Ideal to use when body contact and the effects of substances are experienced as too distressing.

Material
- Washing bowl.
- Bath thermometer.
- Washcloth.
- Towels (To dry off and, if necessary, to put under the bed to protect it from overflowing water).
- Four muslin cloths or two muslin cloths and one pair of warm socks.

A tinkling wash is performed with warm water only, and without the addition of any substances. It can be performed successively on the face, hands, and feet or only on an individual body area. It is ideal for weak, immobile patients, as a clearing and releasing effect can be achieved with little effort on the part of the patient.

Inform the patient about what will happen during the application, and have them lie on their back. A slight elevation of the upper body may be beneficial. During the application, ensure the patient is always covered and only the body region being treated is exposed. To protect the bed from overflowing water, a towel can be placed under the bowl.

First, touch one half of the face with a moistened and wrung-out warm washcloth and let it rest there for a moment. Then repeat the procedure with the other half of the face. Afterwards, both halves of the face are gently dabbed dry with a towel.

Now turn your attention to the patients' hands. Position the bowl on the bed so that the patient can rest their hand inside without effort. To make this more comfortable for the patient, use one of your hands to support their forearm from below. With the other hand, dip into the water and drip the water over the patient's hand. Alternatively, a cloth can be soaked in water and wrung out over the patient's hand. This will produce a tinkling sound, which gives this therapeutic wash its name. This process can be repeated three to five times (Fig. 5.27).

Remove the bowl and gently dab dry the patient's hand, and then wrap in a cloth. Do the same procedure on the other hand. Repeat the sequence on the feet, and cover with socks or wrap in a cloth. During the washing process, it is important that the patient lies comfortably and that the wrist or calf does not lie directly on the edge of the bowl, as this can be uncomfortable.

5.6.3   Oil Dispersion Bath

In an oil dispersion bath, (also sometimes called a "Junge Bath," because of a special oil dispersion device developed by Werner Junge) there is a stable connection between the water and the oil by the means of a special technique whereby oils are atomized. This allows oil to be absorbed through the skin into the blood where it can be metabolized [5]. The heat-storing effect of the oil is thus retained for hours, unlike after a normal bath. This application has a soothing, harmonizing, and enveloping character. It is suitable for patients with depression, physical and mental exhaustion, cardiac arrhythmia, bronchial asthma, and traumatized patients.

5.6.4   Sitting Bath

- *Age Suitability*: as soon as the child can sit on their own.
- *Effects*: depending on substance used (see Chap. 7, Substances).
- *Indications*: depending on substance used (see Chap. 7, Substances).
- *Patient Position*: sitting.
- *Duration*: 5–15 min, 15–20 min post-treatment rest.
- *Note*: The water temperature should be a maximum of 1–2 °C above the patient's body temperature.

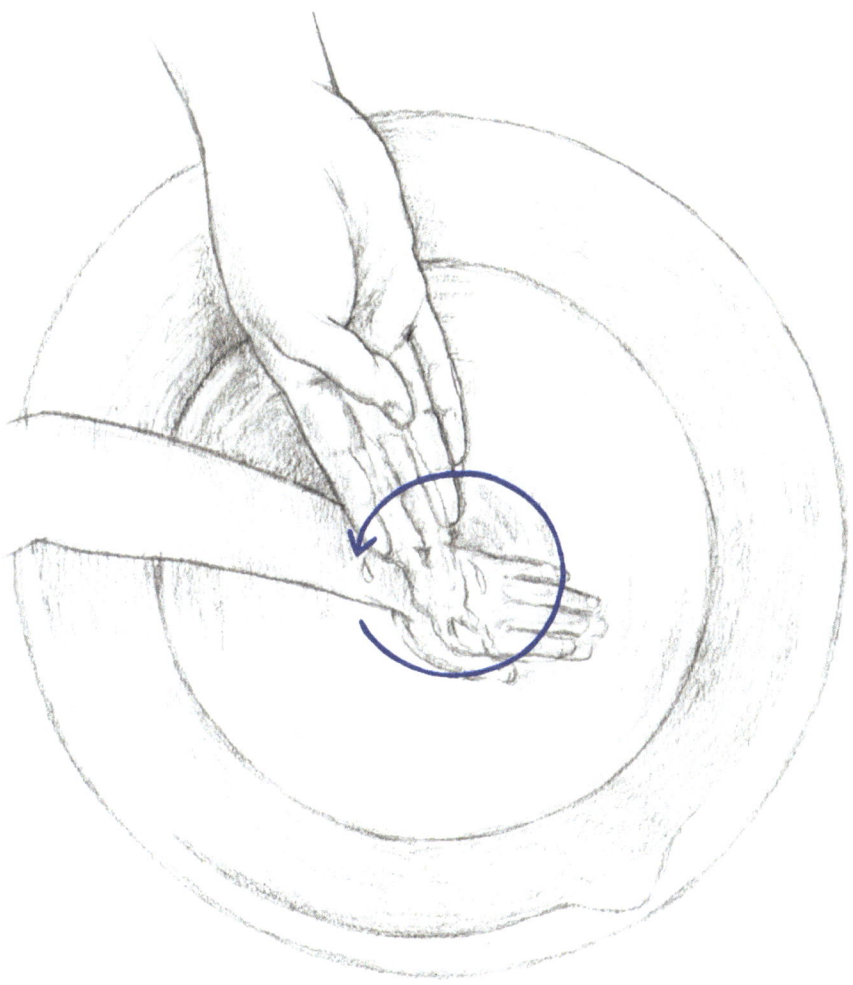

Fig. 5.27 Tinkling wash on the hand

Materials Needed
- Washing bowl/bathtub.
- Bath thermometer.
- Substance (oil, bath milk…).
- Towel (to dry off and, if necessary, to place underneath to soak up the water that has overflowed).

Add the selected substance to the water before the patient is placed in it. Care should be taken to ensure that the water temperature is no more than 1–2 °C above the patient's body temperature.

In a sitting bath, only the patient's lower body is immersed in the water. For younger children, a wash bowl can be used. The child should sit in the bowl with their feet, legs, and upper body remaining out of the water. To protect the patient from cooling down, put socks on their feet and cover their upper body well (Fig. 5.28).

The sitting bath should last 5–15 min, or as long as the patient can comfortably tolerate it. To pass the time, it may be helpful to read the patient a book aloud or tell them a story. Afterwards, dry the lower body well and begin a post-treatment rest period of 15–20 min.

5.6.5 Footbath (with Bath Milk/Oil)

- *Age Suitability*: as soon as the child can sit on their own.
- *Effects*: invigorating, cooling, calming; depending on substance used (see Chap. 7, Substances).
- *Indications*: listlessness, restlessness; depending on substance used (see Chap. 7, Substances).
- *Patient Position*: sitting.
- *Duration*: 5–15 min, 15–20 min post-treatment rest.
- *Note*: The water temperature should be a maximum of 1–2 °C above the patient's body temperature.

Materials Needed
- Wash bowl/foot bath.
- Bath thermometer.
- Substance (oil, bath milk…).
- Towel (for drying and, if necessary, for placing underneath to soak up the over-flowing water).

Mix the selected substance with enough pleasantly warm water (max. 1–2 °C above the patient's body temperature), so that it will reach the patient's ankles. Expose their lower legs to about knee height and place their feet in the water for 5–15 min (Fig. 5.29). Cover their upper legs with a towel to prevent them from cooling down. If the bath water cools down during the application, you can remove the patients' feet and add hot water to return to the initial application temperature.

Dry the feet well and put on socks. Finally, to achieve full effectiveness, the patient should rest for 15–20 min.

5.6.6 Mustard Flour Foot Bath

- *Age Suitability*: from 3 years of age.
- *Effects*: stimulating, releasing, metabolism stimulating, clarifying, warming.
- *Indications*: headache, cold, cystitis, hypotension, cold feet.

Fig. 5.28 Sitting bath

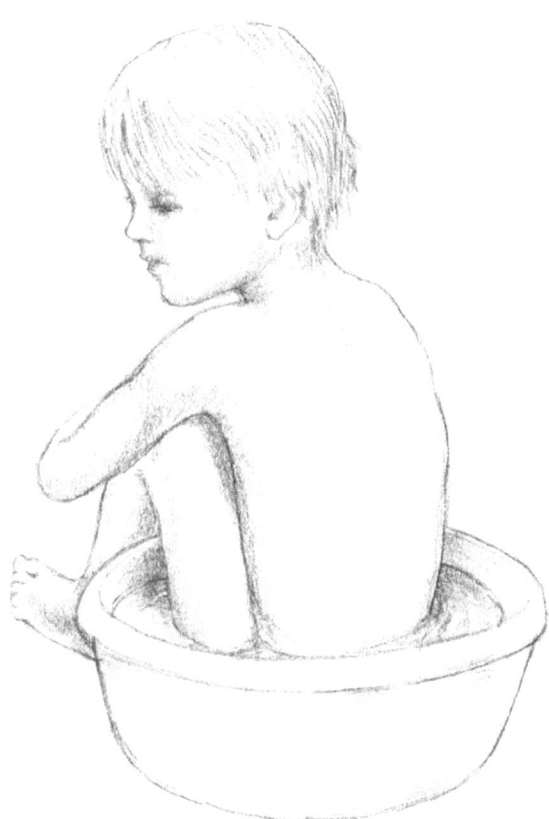

Fig. 5.29 Footbath

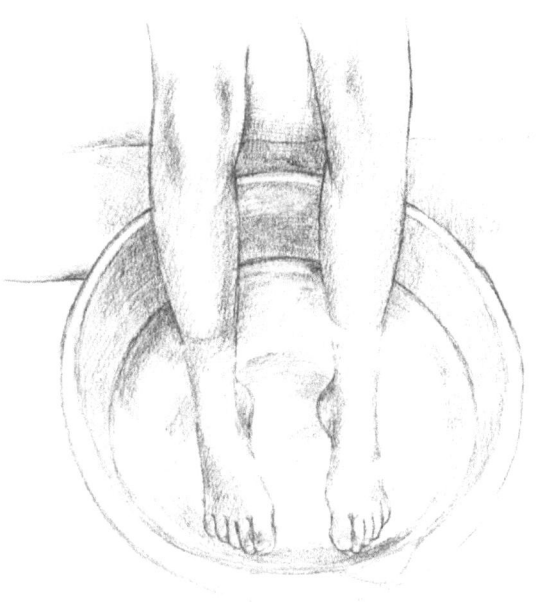

- *Patient Position*: sitting.
- *Duration*: depending on the redness of the skin and the patient's condition, max. 8 min, 15–20 min post-treatment rest.
- *Note*: Prevent contact of the mustard flour with mucous membranes.

Materials Needed
- Wash bowl/foot bath.
- Bath thermometer.
- Black mustard flour (from 3 years: 1 tsp.; from 6 years: 0.5–1 tbsp, from 12 years: 1–2 tbsp black mustard flour).
- Towel (to dry off and, if necessary, to place underneath to soak up the overflowing water).
- Cloth/blanket (to protect the patient from cooling down).
- Nourishing oil.
- Warm socks.

The mustard flour footbath can be highly irritating and can trigger reddening of the skin, which can lead to burns. Avoid contact with mucous membranes. Attentive observation of the skin reaction during the entire application is essential.

The inflammation-like reaction strongly stimulates blood circulation and metabolism. Due to its strong intensity, the mustard flour foot bath should not be used on children under 3 years of age.

Care should be taken to ensure that any reddening of the skin caused by previous foot baths has subsided completely before repeating. Furthermore, the patient and their trusted persons should be informed about the effects before beginning the foot bath. The mustard flour footbath is initially perceived as a tingling sensation and later with a burning sensation. A slight reddening of the skin is desirable.

Mix the mustard flour with enough lukewarm water (37–38 °C) so that it will reach the patients' ankles. Expose the lower legs to about knee height and place the feet in the water. Cover the upper legs with a towel to prevent them from cooling down.

The duration of the foot bath depends on the patient's condition and reddening of their skin, but the maximum time is 8 min.

Afterwards, wash the feet thoroughly with clean water. Ensure that no residue of the mustard flour remains on the foot (pay attention to the spaces between the toes!), as this can lead to burns. Once the feet have been cleaned and dried, rub them with a nourishing oil and put on warm socks.

Afterwards, a rest period of 15–20 min is recommended.

References

1. Batschko E-M (2011) Einführung in die Rhythmischen Einreibungen: Nach Wegmann/Hauschka [Introduction to the rhythmic rubs according to Wegman/Hauschka], 11th edn. Johannes M. Mayer, Stuttgart

2. Findago M (2012) Rhythmic Einreibung: A Handbook from the Ita Wegman Clinic [Therapeutic wraps and compresses, manual from the Ita Wegman clinic], 5th edn. Natura Verlag im Verlag am Goetheanum, Dornach

3. Bächle-Helde B, Bühring U (2014) Heilsame Wickel und Auflagenaus Heilpflanzen, Quark & Co. [Healing compresses and compresses, from medicinal plants, curd & co.] Ulmer Verlag, Bücher

4. Uhlemayr U (2012) Wickel & Co: Bärenstarke Hausmittel für Kinder [Compresses & Co: robust remedies for children], 24th edn. Urs-Verlag, Burgberg

5. Laue B, Salomon A (2009) Kinder natürlich heilen, die besten Hausmittel aus der Apotheke der NatuHealing children naturally, the best home remedies from nature's pharmacy]. Anaconda Verlag GmbH, Cologne

Indications

6

Kira Bindewald and Gisela Blaser

6.1 References

The following table is intended to make it possible to find applications for symptoms/indications that are listed under a different term in the table of contents and therefore cannot be found there.

K. Bindewald (✉)
Department of Pediatric Oncology and Hematology, Charité – Universitätsmedizin Berlin, Berlin, Germany
e-mail: Kira.Bindewald@charite.de

G. Blaser
Bornheim, Germany

Indication	Reference
Loss of appetite under chemotherapy	See oncology > chemotherapy side effects
Abdominal pain	See gastrointestinal diseases/disorders > abdominal cramps, colic
Cystitis	See inflammatory and infectious diseases > urinary tract infection
Bronchitis	See inflammatory and infectious diseases > cough/bronchitis
Bronchitis in newborns, infants	See special applications for premature infants, newborns, infants > cough/bronchitis in newborns, infants
Trouble sleeping through	See mental stress > sleep disorders
Difficulty falling asleep	See mental stress > sleep disorders
Exhaustion due to chemotherapy	See oncology > chemotherapy side effects
Taste disorders due to chemotherapy	See oncology > chemotherapy side effects
Flu infection	See inflammatory and infectious diseases > common cold
Hematoma	See injuries > bruise
Hyperbilirubinemia	See special applications for premature infants, newborns, babies > neonatal jaundice
Icterus	See special applications for premature infants, newborns, babies > neonatal jaundice
Incontinence	See general symptoms > urinary incontinence
Feeling cold	See general symptoms > thermoregulatory disorders
Colic in newborns, infants	See special applications for premature infants, newborns, babies > abdominal cramps, colic in newborns, babies
Meteorism	See gastrointestinal diseases/disorders > flatulence
Meteorism in newborns, infants	See special applications for premature infants, newborns, babies > flatulence in newborns, babies
Constipation in newborns, infants	See special applications for premature infants, newborns, babies > constipation in newborns, babies
Otitis media	See inflammatory and infectious diseases > otitis media
Pneumonia	See inflammatory and infectious diseases > pneumonia
Pneumonia in newborns, infants	See special applications in premature infants, newborns, infants > pneumonia in newborns, infants
Polyneuropathy	See pain > neuropathic pain; general symptoms > paresthesia
Weakness in newborns, infants	See special applications for premature infants, newborns, infants > failure to thrive in newborns, infants
Restlessness, anxious	See psychological stress > anxiety/restlessness
Digestive complaints	See gastrointestinal diseases/disorders > flatulence; > diarrhea; > constipation

6.2   Introduction

The recommendations in this chapter are based on many years of practical experience by nursing professionals. Each external application has been successfully used to supplement and support the therapies prescribed by physicians to treat the symptoms, complaints and/or diseases listed [1–4].

Some general notes in advance:

Although Rhythmic Embrocation is usually recommended as described in Chap. 5, if this specific massage technique has not (yet) been mastered, the applications need not be totally disregarded. Even a simple sensitive massage with one of the recommended preparations can be helpful to the patient.

Both proven ready-to-use preparations, as well as tea infusions and oil mixtures to be prepared by the practitioner themself, are recommended. With many of the applications, there are a number of different substances/preparations to choose from. These options appear in alphabetical order, and are not listed in a way to represent any special priority or weighting. The selection of the respective substance/preparation is left to the discretion of the health caregiver, based on local availability and needs of the respective patient.

The age suitability for each of the applications is based on the experience of nursing professionals and may sometimes differ from the information provided by the manufacturer.

The effect of the preparations usually comes from the essential oils they contain. Premature babies, newborns, infants and toddlers have a particularly keen sense of smell and are sensitive to even the smallest olfactory stimuli. An overstimulation by essential oils should be avoided at all costs; therefore, substances and preparations for certain age groups should be diluted with neutral vegetable oils (so-called base oils such as almond, olive, sesame or possibly sunflower oil). The younger the patient, the higher the dilution required. The respective age-appropriate dosage information can be found with the information about each individual application.

If there is any doubt about the patient's ability to tolerate a preparation with essential oils, applications can be carried out with a neutral vegetable oil (base oil) without additives.

The substances/preparations are described in Chap. 7, Substances, where information on supply sources can also be found.

The following applications, their age suitability and the dosages were made with great care and are based on many years of practitioner experience. However, the authors and the publisher cannot provide any guarantee or be held liable for the effectiveness or safety of any applications or therapies described herein.

6.3 Special Applications for Premature Infants, Newborns and Babies

6.3.1 Respiratory Distress Syndrome/Infant Respiratory Distress Syndrome (IRDS) in Preterm Infants

Recommended for use in cases of *bradycardia* as well as "floppiness" in premature infants, newborns, babies.

Application
Rosemary Socks, see Chap. 5.5.11.

Substance/Preparation
Rosemary ointment 1% (Rosemary ointment in the concentration of 1% is not commercially available as a ready-to-use preparation and must be specially prepared in the pharmacy.)

Effect
Invigorating, strengthening, vitalizing.

Age Suitability
Premature infants (from 28 weeks), newborns, infants.

Instructions
Apply Rosemary Socks as described in Chap. 5.5.11.

Frequency
1 time daily, preferably in the morning before noon. If used later in the day, the stimulating effect of rosemary may cause sleep disturbances in the evening.

Contraindication
Allergy to rosemary (Rosmarini aetheroleum).

Note
For use in premature babies, infants and young children up to 2 years of age, the concentration of rosemary oil in the ointment must not exceed **1%,** because, at higher concentrations, there is a risk of laryngeal spasm. Therefore, the commercially available rosemary ointment 10% must not be used under any circumstances.

6.3.2   Abdominal Cramps, Colic in Newborns, Infants

The following applications are also recommended in cases of *flatulence (meteorism), constipation* in newborns and infants.

Application (1)
One-Handed Abdominal Circles for Infants, see Chap. 5.4.5.

Substance/Preparation
Melissa oil, ready-to-use preparation (Wala).

Effect
Antispasmodic, decongestant, analgesic, sedative.

Age Suitability
All ages; dosage is based on the age of the patient.

Dosage
0–12 months: Dilute the melissa oil with equal parts (1:1) almond or olive oil, or sunflower oil as a substitute.
    From 1 year of age: Undiluted melissa oil can be used.

Instructions
Using an age-appropriate dosage, rub/massage 2–3 ml of the oil into the abdomen as described in Chap. 5.4.5. Avoid putting pressure on the bladder. Allow for a 15–30 minutes (min.). Post-treatment rest.

Frequency
If necessary, several times a day, not directly following a meal (approx. 30 min. interval).

Contraindications
Acute abdomen.
    Allergy/intolerance to an ingredient of the preparation, as listed in the instructions for use/content information.

Application (2)
Warm (Moist) Wrapped Compress for the abdomen, see Chap. 5.5.2.

Substance/Preparation
Oxalis essence, ready-to-use premixed preparation (Wala).

Effect
Antispasmodic, decongestant, analgesic, sedative.

Age Suitability
All ages, dosage is based on the age of the patient.

Dosage
0–12 months: ½ tsp. oxalis essence to 250 ml water.
    From 1 year of age: 1 tsp. oxalis essence to 250 ml water.
    From 2 years of age: 1 tbsp oxalis essence to 250 ml water.

Instructions
Mix an age-appropriate dosage of the oxalis essence with 250 ml of warm (40 °C) water. Prepare the wrapped compress as described in Chap. 5.5.2. Allow for 15–30 min. Post-treatment rest.

Frequency
12 times per day.

Contraindications
Acute abdomen, inflammation or injury of the skin in the treated area. Allergy/ intolerance to one of the ingredients of the preparation, as listed in the instructions for use.

6.3.3 Flatulence (Meteorism) in Newborns, Infants

For recommendations, see Abdominal cramps, colic in newborns, infants.

6.3.4 Bradycardia in Preterm Infants

For recommendations, see respiratory distress syndrome/Infant respiratory distress syndrome (IRDS) in preterm infants.

6.3.5 Weak Constitution in Newborns, Infants

Application
Rhythmic Embrocation for Infants (Warming Breaths), see Chap. 5.4.3.

Substance/Preparation
Mallow oil, ready-to-use preparation (Wala).

Effect
Enveloping, warming, relaxing.

Age Suitability
From neonatal age; dosage depends on the age of the patient.

Dosage
0–12 months: Dilute the mallow oil with equal parts (1:1) of a neutral oil (almond or olive oil, alternatively sunflower oil).
    From 1 year of age the mallow oil preparation can be used undiluted.

Instructions
Using an age-appropriate dosage, rub/massage in 2–3 ml of the oil using the method described in Chap. 5.4.3. Allow for 15–30 min. post-treatment rest. During the embrocation and following rest period, take extra care to ensure the patient is kept warm.

Frequency
1–2 times daily.

Contraindications
Allergy/intolerance to an ingredient of the preparation, as listed in the instructions for use/content information.

6.3.6 Cough/Bronchitis in Newborns, Infants

The following application is also recommended for **pneumonia** in newborns, and infants.

Application
Farmer's Cheese (Quark) rapped Compress, (warm) for the chest, see Chap. 5.5.7.

Substance/Preparation
Farmer's cheese (quark), preferably lean (without additives).

Effect
Relaxing for spasmodic cough, expectorant, respiratory deepening.

Age Suitability
From 1 month.
    All patients beyond infancy.

Instructions
Prepare and apply the warm chest compress with farmer's cheese (quark) as described in Chap. 5.5.7. The compress should remain in place for 2–3 h. If necessary, it can also be left on overnight.

Frequency
1x per day, preferably in the evening.

Contraindications
Neurodermatitis, cow milk allergy.

Note
Because the compress is applied centrally, the farmer's cheese (quark) must be warmed to 36–37 °C (body temperature) as described in Chap. 5.5.7. Otherwise, there is a risk that the patient will cool down.

6.3.7 Pneumonia (Pneumonia) in Newborns, Infants

For recommendations, see Bronchitis in newborns, infants.

6.3.8   Mottled, Cool Skin in Premature Infants

Application
Rhythmic embrocation for Infants (Warming Breaths), full body or partial, see Chap. 5.4.3.

Substance/Preparation
Mallow oil, ready-to-use premixed preparation (Wala).

Effect
Warming, enveloping, relaxing.

Age Suitability
Premature infants (from 28 weeks); also newborns and infants; dosage depends on the age of the patient.

Dosage
Premature infants: Dilute the mallow oil preparation with 2 parts (1:2) base oil (neutral oil), e.g., almond or olive oil, alternatively sunflower oil (1 part mallow oil to 2 parts base oil).

Newborns and infants up to 12 months: Dilute the mallow oil preparation with equal parts (1:1) almond or olive oil, alternatively sunflower oil.

From 1 year of age the mallow oil preparation can be used undiluted.

Instructions
Using an age-appropriate dosage, rub/massage in 2–3 ml of the oil using the method described in Chap. 5.4.3 allow for 15–30 min. post-treatment rest. During the embrocation and following rest period, take extra care to ensure the patient is kept warm.

Frequency
1 time per day.

Contraindications
Intolerance/allergy to an ingredient of the preparation according to the instructions for use/content information.

Notes
For premature infants in incubators: Use only low-concentration oil to avoid sensory overload. Ready-to-use preparations must be diluted with almond or olive oil, or alternatively sunflower oil, in a ratio of 1:2, or if necessary 1:3 or more. As an alternative, use pure almond, olive or sunflower oil (without additives) for the embrocation.

Mottled, cool skin is an expression of a thermoregulatory disorder. Take care with regard to clothing, bedding and ambient temperature to ensure that the patient neither cools down nor builds up heat.

6.3.9 "Floppiness" in Premature Infants

For recommendations, see Respiratory distress syndrome/Infant respiratory distress syndrome (IRDS) in preterm infants.

6.3.10 Constipation (Obstipation) in Newborns, Infants

For recommendations, see Abdominal cramps, colic in newborns, infants.

6.4 General Symptoms

6.4.1 Exhaustion/Exhaustive States

The following applications are also recommended for *listlessness* and *general weakness*.

Application (1)
Rhythmic Embrocation:

- Rhythmic Embrocation for Infants (Warming Breaths), see Chaps. 5.4.3–5.4.5
- Back Embrocation, see Chap. 5.3.6
  Two-Handed Abdominal Embrocation, see Chap. 5.3.8
- Diamond Formation Embrocation see Chap. 5.3.7
- Foot Embrocation, see Chap. 5.3.13.

Each embrocation can be performed individually or in combination with the others. When combined, patients (beyond infancy) should be worked on from their center outward toward their periphery.

Substance/Preparation
Mallow oil, ready-to-use preparation (Wala), especially recommended for back and foot as well as whole-body embrocation for infants, or melissa oil, ready-to-use preparation (Wala), especially recommended for abdominal embrocation, orSolum oil, ready-to-use preparation (Wala), especially recommended for back and foot embrocation.

Effect
Mild warming, enveloping, restorative, strengthening.

Age Suitability
All ages, dosage is based on the age of the patient.

Dosage
0–12 months: Dilute the selected preparation with equal parts (1:1) neutral oil (almond or olive oil, alternatively sunflower oil).

From 1 year of age, each of the preparations can be used undiluted.

Instructions
Using an age-appropriate dosage, rub/massage in 2–3 ml of the oil using the method described in Chap. 5.3, 5.4. Allow for 15–30 min. post-treatment rest. During the embrocation and following rest period, take extra care to ensure the patient is kept warm.

Frequency
1–2 times per day as needed; in the morning the application has a rather invigorating effect, in the evening it has a relaxing and sleep-promoting effect.

Contraindications
The abdominal embrocation should not be used in cases of intestinal obstruction or bleeding in the abdominal area.

Allergy/intolerance to an ingredient of the preparation, as listed in the instructions for use/content information.

Note
The two-handed abdominal embrocation can also be performed with one hand. In this case, apply the oil to the abdomen using 3–5 circular movements in a clockwise direction, starting from the right groin. In the case of tumors or metastases in the abdomen, the embrocation should be particularly gentle.

Application (2)
Oil Compress—for abdomen, see Chap. 5.5.1.

Substance/Preparation
Melissa oil, ready-to-use preparation (Wala) or solum oil, ready-to-use preparation (Wala).

Effect
Stimulates the building metabolism, strengthening, warming.

Age Suitability
All ages, dosage is based on the age of the patient.

Dosage

0–12 months: dilute the selected preparation with equal parts (1:1) neutral oil (almond or olive oil, alternatively sunflower oil).

From 1 year of age, any preparation can be used undiluted.

Instructions

Using age-appropriate dosage, apply one of the selected oils to the abdomen, as described in Chap. 5.5.1.

Frequency

1–2 times a day as needed; in the morning the application has an invigorating effect, in the evening it has a relaxing and sleep-promoting effect.

Since there is no evaporative cooling effect, the compress can also be left for a longer period, for example overnight.

Contraindications

Unclear abdomen, skin defects in the area of application, inflammatory processes, fever.

Allergy/intolerance to an ingredient of the preparation, as listed in the instructions for use/content information.

Application (3)

Footbath, see Chap. 5.6.5.

Substance/Preparation

Rosemary Activating Bath, ready-to-use preparation (Weleda).

Effect

Builds up, strengthens, stabilizes circulation.

Age Suitability

From 6 years of age, the dosage depends on the age of the patient.

Dosage

From 6 years of age: ½ cap bath milk.

From 12 years: 1 cap bath milk.

Instructions

Prepare and carry out the footbath as described in Chap. 5.6.5. To have an invigorating effect, the water temperature should not be higher than 36–37 °C. Using a footbath tub is recommended. For children up to approx. 12 years of age, the water should only reach ankle height; for adolescents, the lower legs can be immersed up to the middle of the calves.

After the footbath, prevent the feet from cooling down with socks/stockings made of natural materials (wool, cotton, silk). A post-treatment rest period is not necessary, the patient can and *should* move.

Frequency
1 time per day, preferably in the morning before noon. If used later in the day, the stimulating effect of rosemary may cause sleep disturbances in the evening.

Contraindications
Skin lesions in the area of application; arterial hypertension Allergy/intolerance to an ingredient of the preparation, as listed in the instructions for use/content information.

6.4.2   Urinary Incontinence, e.g. After Removal of a Permanent Catheter

For recommendations, see Urinary tract infection.

6.4.3   Urinary Retention

For recommendations, see Urinary tract infection.

6.4.4   Insect Bite

For recommendations, see Itching.

6.4.5   Cold Legs and Feet

Application (1)
Rhythmic Embrocation:Back Embrocation, see Chap. 5.3.6 Two-Handed Knee Circles, see Chap. 5.3.11 Two-Handed Calf Embrocation, see Chap. 5.3.12 Foot Embrocation, see Chap. 5.3.13.

Each embrocation can be performed alone or in combination with the others. When combined, patients should be worked on from their center outward toward their periphery.

Substance/Preparation
Cuprum metallicum praep. 0.4% ointment, ready-to-use preparation (Weleda) or Copper ointment red, ready-to-use preparation (Wala) or Lavender relaxing care oil, ready-to-use preparation (Weleda) or Solum oil, ready-to-use preparation (Wala).

Note

Cuprum metallicum praep. 0.4% ointment and copper ointment red may be used for foot embrocation only. Lavender and Solum oil may be used for any of the partial embrocation mentioned above.

Age Suitability

From 1 year of age: Lavender Relaxing Care Oil; Solum Oil.

From 3 years of age: Cuprum metallicum praep. 0.4% ointment; copper ointment red.

Instructions

Using an age-appropriate dosage, rub/massage in 2–3 ml of the selected oil using the method described in Chap. 5.3. Following the embrocation, the feet should be kept warm with socks/stockings made of natural materials (wool, cotton, silk) and the patient should be encouraged to move.

Frequency

1 time per day, preferably in the morning; if necessary, it can also be used in the evening before bedtime.

Contraindications

Intolerance/allergy to an ingredient of the preparation used according to the instructions for use/content information.

Note

Cuprum metallicum praep. 0.4% ointment and copper ointment should not be applied on large areas, as their strong heat-generating effect could lead to overheating of the organism and increase of blood pressure.

Application (2)

Mustard Flour Footbath, see Chap. 5.6.6.

Substance/Preparation

Black mustard flour (Semen Sinapis nigrae pulv.)

Effect

Promotes blood circulation, stimulates the metabolism, draining.

Age Suitability

From 3 years of age, the dosage depends on the age of the patient.

Dosage

From 3 years of age: 1 tsp. black mustard flour to approx. 5 liters of water.

From 6 years of age: 0.5–1 tbsp black mustard flour to approx. 5 liters of water.

From 12 years of age: 1–2 tbsp black mustard flour to approx. 5 liters of water.

Instructions
Prepare the footbath according to the age dosage and perform as described in Chap. 5.6.6. After a rest phase, the patient should be encouraged to move.

Frequency
The application should be carried out for 5 days followed by a break of 2 days; this sequence should be continued for another 2 weeks.

If necessary, this 3-week treatment series can be repeated after a break of 3 weeks.

Contraindications
Skin lesions in the area of application.
Mustard flour intolerance/allergy.

Note
If the skin in the foot area is still very red the day after a mustard flour footbath, the next one should only be carried out when the redness has faded.

Application (3)
Footbath, see Chap. 5.6.5.

Substance/Preparation
Rosemary Activating Bath, ready-to-use preparation (Weleda).

Age Suitability
From 6 years, the dosage depends on the age of the patient.

Dosage
From 6 years of age: ½ cap bath milk.
From 12 years of age: 1 cap bath milk.

Instructions for the Footbath
Prepare and carry out the footbath as described in Chap. 5.6.5. To have an invigorating effect, the water temperature should not be higher than 36–37 °C. Using a footbath tub is recommended. For children up to approx. 12 years of age, the water should only reach ankle height; for adolescents, the lower legs can be immersed up to the middle of the calves. Following the footbath, prevent the feet from cooling with socks/stockings made of natural materials (wool, cotton, silk). A post-treatment rest period is not necessary, the patient can and should move.

Frequency
1 time daily, preferably in the morning before noon. If used later in the day, the stimulating effect of rosemary may cause sleep disturbances in the evening.

Contraindications
Skin lesions in the area of application, hypertensionRosemary intolerance/allergy.

Effect
The applications (1), (2) and (3) have a lasting effect on circulation and warming.

Other Applications (4)
For a general feeling of cold, shivering, susceptibility to infections, see Thermoregulation Disorders.

6.4.6   Palliative Care—Accompanying Applications

Application (1)
Rhythmic Embrocation:

- Hand Embrocation, see Chap. 5.3.9.
- Foot Embrocation, see Chap. 5.3.13.
- or Figure Eights for the Foot, see Chap. 5.3.14,
- Pentagram Embrocation, see Chap. 5.3.15.

Each embrocation can be performed alone or in combination with the others. Before the pentagram embrocation, cold feet should be warmed with an embrocation using Solum oil.

Substances/Preparations
Aurum/Lavandula comp. Cream, ready-to-use preparation (Weleda) or Solum oil, ready-to-use preparation (Wala), especially recommended for foot embrocation.

Age Suitability and Dosage
0–12 months: Solum oil, mixed in equal parts (1:1) with a neutral oil (almond or olive oil; alternatively sunflower oil).
From 1 year of age: Aurum/Lavandula comp. Cream; Solum oil (undiluted).

Instructions
Using an age-appropriate dosage, rub/massage in 2–3 ml of the oil, or an approx. Pea-sized amount of Aurum/Lavandula comp. Cream, using the method described in Chap. 5.3. During the embrocation and following rest period, take extra care to ensure the patient is kept warm.

Frequency
Hand, foot embrocation 2–3 times a day.
Pentagram embrocation 1 time a day.

Contraindications

Do not conduct a hand embrocation if the patient has a tendency toward epileptic seizures.

Intolerance/allergy to an ingredient of the selected preparation according to the instructions for use/content information.

Application (2)

Heart Compress with Ointment.

Substance/Preparation

Aurum/Lavandula comp. Cream, ready-to-use preparation (Weleda).

Age Suitability

From 2 years of age (for an alternative for infants and younger children, see "Note").

Preparation and Instructions for Implementation

Materials Needed

- Substance Cloth, use a cloth handkerchief or other thin cloth made of cotton or linen approx. 12 x 12 cm.
- Outer Wrap, use a cotton or wool cloth.
- Wooden spatula or plastic knife.
- Aurum/Lavandula comp. Cream.
- Hot-water bottle.

Using the spatula/knife, apply a thin layer of the ointment to the substance cloth to create a shiny (mirrored) surface. Slightly warm the ointment pad on a hot-water bottle or heater before placing it on the heart region of the chest; the outer cloth can be used to wrap the chest. The compress should be left in place for at least an hour, but can also be left on overnight. After use, the substance cloth can be stored in a plastic bag, ointment can be reapplied and the cloth reused.

Frequency

1 time per day, preferably in the evening.

Contraindications

Intolerance/allergy to ingredients of the preparation used according to the instructions for use/content information.

Note

For children 0–2 years of age, instead of using the heart compress, apply a small amount of Aurum/Lavandula comp. Ointment very thinly to the skin and gently massaged in.

Effect

The applications (1) and (2) have a calming, relaxing, warming and relieving effect in the dying process.

Application (3)
Tinkling Wash, see Chap. 5.6.2.

Substance
Water, warm (37–38 °C).

Effect
Soothing, clarifying, releasing.

Age Suitability
From approx. 10 years of age.

Instructions
The tinkling wash is performed as described in Chap. 5.6.2.

Frequency
1 time daily.

Contraindications
None known.

6.4.7 Paresthesia

Application (1)
Oil Compress—for the area of paresthesia, see Chap. 5.5.1.

Substance/Preparation
Aconite pain oil, ready-to-use preparation (Wala) or Solum oil, ready-to-use preparation (Wala).

Effect
Balancing, soothing, analgesic.

Age Suitability
From 1 year of age: Solum oil.
   From 6 years of age: Aconite pain oil.

Instructions
Prepare the compress with the selected oil (note age suitability) and apply to the affected area as described in Chap. 5.5.1. If the compress is applied to the extremities, a large outer towel is not required. In the case of application to the torso, a towel or scarf is sufficient for wrapping.

Frequency
1–2 times a day.

As there is no evaporative cooling effect, the compress can be left on for a longer period of time, even overnight.

Contraindications
Skin defects in the area of application.

Allergy/intolerance to an ingredient of the preparation, as listed in the instructions for use/content information.

Note
Aconite pain oil is highly potent and should be dosed carefully.

Application (2)
Rhythmic Embrocation of the affected area or—if the affected area is sensitive to touch or difficult to access—a combination of: Back Embrocation, see sect. 5.3.6 and Two-Handed Abdominal Embrocation, see sect. 5.3.8 and Foot Embrocation, see sect. 5.3.13.

Substance/Preparation
Aconite pain oil, ready-to-use preparation (Wala)—for back or extremity embrocation—or.

Melissa oil, ready-to-use preparation (Wala)—for abdomen and feet embrocation—or.

Solum oil, ready-to-use preparation (Wala)—for all body areas.

Age Suitability
From 1 year: Melissa oil, Solum oil.

From 6 years: Aconite pain oil.

Instructions
Take note of the age suitability when selecting oil. Rub/massage in 2–3 ml of the oil (or a quantity corresponding to the treated area) as described in Chap. 5.3.

Frequency
1–2 times a day.

Contraindications
Skin defects in the area of application.

Allergy/intolerance to an ingredient of the preparation, as listed in the instructions for use/content information.

Note
Aconite pain oil is highly potent and should be dosed carefully.

Effect

The applications (1) and (2) have a balancing, relaxing, analgesic, enveloping effect.

6.4.8 Irritable Bladder

For recommendations, see Urinary tract infection.

6.4.9 Convalescence Phase

For example, after:

- Surviving a disease
- Chemotherapy
- Radiotherapy.

Application (1)
Rhythmic Embrocation:

- Back Embrocation, see Chap. 5.3.6.
- Two-Handed Abdominal Embrocation, see Chap. 5.3.8.
- Foot Embrocation, see Chap. 5.3.13.

Each embrocation can be performed alone or in combination with the others. When combined, patients should be worked on from their center outward toward their periphery. Especially with newborns and infants, an embrocation that induces warming breath can be used, see Chap. 5.4.3.

Substance/Preparation
Mallow oil, ready-to-use preparation (Wala).

Effect
Relaxing, mildly warming, enveloping, mood-lifting, reassuring.

Age Suitability
All ages, dosage is based on the age of the patient.

Dosage
0–12 months: Dilute the mallow oil with equal parts (1:1) neutral oil (almond or olive oil, alternatively sunflower oil).
From 1 year of age, the mallow oil can be used undiluted.

Instructions of the Embrocation

Using an age-appropriate dosage, rub/massage in 2–3 ml of the oil, or a quantity of the oil corresponding to the treated body areas, using the method described in Chap. 5.3/5.4. Allow for 20–30 min. Post-treatment rest. During the embrocation and following rest period, take extra care to ensure the patient is kept warm.

Frequency

1–2 times per day.

Contraindications

Allergy/intolerance to an ingredient of the preparation, as listed in the instructions for use/content information.

Application (2)

Warm (Moist) Wrapped Compress—for liver, see Chap. 5.5.2.

Substance/Preparation

Yarrow (Millefolii herba), tea drug.

Effect

Builds and strengthens by stimulating liver function.

Age Suitability

From 3 years of age, the dosage depends on the age of the patient.

Dosage

From 3 years of age: ½ tsp. tea drug.
> From 6 years of age: 1 tsp. tea drug.
> From 12 years of age: 1 tbsp. Tea drug.

Preparation and Instructions

Pour 300 ml of boiling water over (an age-appropriate dosage of) the yarrow herb and leave it to infuse for 3–5 min. Strain and let cool at room temperature for another 10 min, so that it reaches an application temperature of about 60 °C.

Use this infusion to prepare and apply the compress as described in Chap. 5.5.2.

A hot-water bottle with approx. 60 °C warm water (mix 2/3 boiling hot water with 1/3 cold water) can be placed on the outer wrap to avoid cooling. After 20–30 min., remove the moist substance and middle cloths, before tightly reclosing the outer layer. During the post-treatment rest period of approx. 30 min, the hot-water bottle can remain in place.

Frequency

1 time per day, preferably after lunch with approx. 30 min. Interval between meals.

Contraindications
Unclear abdomen, skin defects in the area of application, inflammatory processes, fever, intolerance/allergy to yarrow.

6.4.10 Weakness, General

For application recommendations, see Exhaustion/Exhaustive states.

6.4.11 Thermoregulation Disorders

For example: constant feeling of cold, shivering, sensitivity to cold, susceptibility to infections.

Application (1)
Wrapped Ginger Compress—for kidney, see Chap. 5.5.5.

Substance/Preparation
Ginger powder.

Age Suitability
From 2 years of age, the dosage depends on the age of the patient.

Dosage
From 2 years of age: ½ tsp. ginger powder to 300–400 ml water.
    From 6 years of age: 1 tsp. ginger powder to 300–400 ml water.
    From 12 years of age: 1 tbsp ginger powder to 300–400 ml water.

Instructions
Using an age-appropriate dosage, prepare and apply the wrapped ginger compress as described in Chap. 5.5.5. The kidney area (right and left of the lumbar spine in the area of the lower ribs) should be well covered by the substance cloth.

Frequency
1 time per day, preferably in the morning or early afternoon before 15:00 h; application later in the day may cause sleep disturbances due to the stimulating effect of ginger. Note: redness from previous treatments must have clearly subsided before the next application is carried out.

Apply for 5 days, followed by a 2-day break; this sequence should be repeated for another 2 weeks. If necessary, the treatment series can be repeated after a 3-week break.

Contraindications
Fever, kidney-related (renal) hypertension, sensitive skin, injury, acute inflammation or sensory disturbance in the area of application. Intolerance/allergy to ginger.

Note
Ginger can irritate the skin; patients must remain under observation during the entire application. If the irritation is too intense, stop the treatment before the end of the recommended treatment time.

During application, the feet should be warm or kept warm with a good covering, or if required, with socks (made of natural material such as wool, cotton, silk) or a hot-water bottle (not in cases of sensitivity disorders of legs/feet).

Application (2)
Warm (Moist) Wrapped Compress—for abdomen, see Chap. 5.5.2.

Substance/Preparation
Chamomile flowers (Matricariae flos), tea drug.

Age Suitability
From 3 years of age, the dosage depends on the age of the patient.

Dosage
From 3 years of age: ½ tsp. tea drug.
   From 6 years of age: 1 tsp. tea drug.
   From 12 years of age: 1 tbsp tea drug.

Preparation and Instructions
Pour 300 ml of boiling water over (an age-appropriate dosage of) the chamomile flowers and leave it to infuse for 3–5 min. Strain and let cool at room temperature for another 10 min, so that it reaches an application temperature of about 60 °C.

Use this infusion to prepare the compress and apply as described in Chap. 5.5.2.

A hot water bottle with approx. 60 ° C warm water (mix 2/3 boiling hot water with 1/3 cold water) can be placed on the outer layer to prevent cooling. After 10–25 min., remove the moist substance and middle cloths, before tightly reclosing the outer layer. During the post-treatment rest period of approx. 30 min, the hot-water bottle can remain in place.

Frequency
1 time per day.

Apply for 5 days, followed by a 2-day break; this sequence should be repeated for another 2 weeks. If necessary, the treatment series can be repeated after a 3-week break.

Contraindications

Unclear abdomen, skin defects in the area of application, inflammatory processes, fever.

Allergy/intolerance to chamomile.

Note

During application, the feet should be warm or kept warm with a good covering, or if required, with socks (made of natural material such as wool, cotton, silk) or a hot-water bottle (not in cases of sensitivity disorders of legs/feet).

Effect

The applications (1) and (2) sustainably stimulate the body's own heat production.

Other Applications (3)

If there is a tendency to have cold feet, see Cold Legs and Feet.

6.4.12 Tension, Muscular

For recommendations to ease muscular tension, e.g., in the shoulder-neck area, in the back area and the associated complaints, see Pain in the Musculoskeletal System.

6.5   Inflammatory and Infectious Diseases

6.5.1   Bronchial Asthma

For recommendations, see Bronchitis, obstructive.

6.5.2   Bronchitis, Obstructive

The following recommendations also apply to **Bronchial asthma.**

Application (1)

Wrapped with Ginger Compress for Chest, see Chap. 5.5.5.

For seizure prevention during *symptom-free* intervals.

Substance/Preparation

Ginger powder.

Effect

Warming, relaxing, respiratory deepening, expectorant.

Age Suitability
From 2 years of age, the dosage depends on the age of the patient.

Dosage
From 2 years of age: 1/2 tsp. ginger powder to 300–400 ml water.
    From 6 years of age: 1 tsp. ginger powder to 300–400 ml water.
    From 12 years of age: 1 tbsp ginger powder to 300–400 ml water.

Instructions
Prepare and apply wrapped ginger compress to the chest as described in Chap. 5.5.5.

Frequency
1 time per day, preferably in the morning or early afternoon before 15:00 h; application later in the day may cause sleep disturbances due to the stimulating effect of ginger. Note: redness from previous treatments must have clearly subsided before the next application is carried out.

Apply for 5 days, followed by a 2-day break; this sequence should be repeated for another 2 weeks. If necessary, the treatment series can be repeated after a 3-week break.

Contraindications
Fever, injured skin, acute inflammation and/or sensory disturbances in the area of application.
    Intolerance/allergy to ginger.

Note
If the nipples will have contact with the ginger compress, smear them with petroleum jelly or an oil-based cream without irritants for protection and cover them with gauze or a cotton pad.

Ginger can irritate the skin; patients must remain under observation during the entire application. If the irritation is too intense, stop the treatment before the end of the recommended treatment time.

Application (2)
For seizure prevention during *symptom-free* intervals –.
    Ginger Compress—for the kidneys, see Chap. 5.5.5.
    This application is particularly suitable if the chest compress is not well tolerated and/or if the patient is prone to cold hands and feet.

Substance/Preparation
Ginger powder.

Age Suitability
From 2 years of age, the dosage depends on the age of the patient.

Dosage

From 2 years of age: 1/2 tsp. ginger powder to 300–400 ml water.
   From 6 years of age: 1 tsp. ginger powder to 300–400 ml water.
   From 12 years of age: 1 tbsp ginger powder to 300–400 ml water.

Instructions

Using an age-appropriate dosage, prepare and apply the ginger wrap as described in Chap. 5.5.5. The kidney area (right and left of the lumbar spine in the area of the lower ribs) should be well covered by the inner cloth (substance cloth).

Frequency

1 time per day, preferably in the morning or early afternoon before 15:00 h; application later in the day may cause sleep disturbances due to the stimulating effect of ginger. Note: redness from previous treatments must have clearly subsided before the next application is carried out.

Apply for 5 days, followed by a 2-day break; this sequence should be repeated for another 2 weeks. If necessary, the treatment series can be repeated after a 3-week break.

Contraindications

Fever, kidney-related (renal) hypertension, sensitive skin, injury, acute inflammation or sensory disturbance in the area of application. Intolerance/allergy to ginger.

Note

Ginger can irritate the skin; patients must remain under observation during the entire application. If the irritation is too intense, stop the treatment before the end of the recommended treatment time.

During application, the feet should be warm or kept warm with a good covering, or if required, with socks (made of natural material such as wool, cotton, silk) or a hot-water bottle (not in cases of sensitivity disorders of legs/feet).

Application (3)

In the event of respiratory distress, in addition to medication prescribed by a doctor.
   Rhythmic Embrocation:

- Good Night Figure Eights, see Chap. 5.3.6.
- Calf Embrocation, see Chap. 5.3.12.
- Foot Embrocation, see Chap. 5.3.13.

When combining the above embrocations, patients should be worked on from their center outward toward their periphery. In the case of younger patients, instead of an embrocation or following it, sit the child on your lap and simply hold their feet, gently enveloping them to release the tension from their airways.

Substance/Preparation
Base oil (neutral oil), e.g., almond or olive oil, alternatively sunflower oil—especially for calf and foot embrocation—or copper ointment red, ready-to-use preparation (Wala)—intense warming effect, especially suitable for cold in the back area and tendency to cold feet for figure eight in the kidney area and foot embrocation.

Effect
Tension relieving, calming, antispasmodic, warming.

Age Suitability
From 1 year: embrocation with a base oil.
   From 3 years: embrocation with copper ointment red.

Instructions
Take note of the age suitability when selecting a substance. Rub/massage in 2–3 ml of the oil (or a quantity corresponding to the treated area) as described in Chap. 5.3.
   Note: Copper ointment red is highly potent and must be dosed very carefully. For foot embrocation, a pea-sized amount per foot is sufficient; only slightly more is required for a figure eight.

Contraindications
When using copper ointment red: hypersensitivity/allergy to copper oxide, hypertension, fever.

Note
In obstructive respiratory diseases, the use of essential oils should be avoided to prevent irritation of the respiratory tract. Use neutral oils (base oils) without additives for the applications.

6.5.3   Cold

The following application is recommended when a cold is imminent, as well as for *colds, headaches, sinusitis, and maxillary sinusitis.*
   Additional recommendations for symptoms such as cough, sore throat, earache can be found under the respective symptom in the table of contents.

Application
Mustard Flour Footbath, see Chap. 5.6.6.

Substance/Preparation
Black mustard flour (Semen Sinapis nigrae pulv.)

Effect
Promotes blood circulation, stimulates metabolism, draining.

Age Suitability
From 3 years of age, the dosage depends on the age of the patient.

Dosage
From 3 years of age: 1 tsp. black mustard flour to approx. 5 liters of water.
    From 6 years of age: 0.5–1 tbsp black mustard flour to approx. 5 liters of water.
    From 12 years of age: 1–2 tbsp black mustard flour to approx. 5 liters of water.

Instructions
Noting age-appropriate dosage, prepare and carry out the footbath as described in Chap. 5.6.5.

Frequency
1 time daily.

Contraindications
Skin lesions in the area of application.
    Mustard flour intolerance/allergy.

Note
A mustard flour footbath may even be used in cases of mild fever, as it helps the body to release excess heat.

6.5.4 Fever

Application (1)
Therapeutic Whole Body Wash, see Chap. 5.6.1.

Substance/Preparation
Peppermint (Mentha piperita), tea drug.

Effect
Reduction of body temperature by 0.5 to 1 °C; refreshment and well-being.

Age Suitability
From 6 years of age, the dosage depends on the age of the patient.

Dosage
From 6 years of age: 1 tbsp tea drug.
    From 12 years of age: 2 tbsp tea drug.

Instructions

Pour 500 ml of boiling water over (an age-appropriate dosage of) the dried peppermint leaves and leave it to infuse for 5–10 min. Strain and then mix infusion with 3–4 liters of water to reach a temperature 1–2 °C below the patient's body temperature.

Starting with the arms and legs, wash the skin with a thoroughly wet washcloth, then move on to the torso. Lightly dab the skin and do not dry. The evaporative process, together with the menthol from the peppermint, has a cooling effect on the skin.

Frequency

Can be performed anytime there is an onset of fever after confirming that the patient is uniformly warm over the entire body, including hands and feet. There must be no systematic fever.

Contraindication

Allergy to peppermint.

Note

For children, do not use peppermint oil: It can cause glottic spasms and is too cold for children.

Application (2)

Therapeutic Whole Body Wash, see Chap. 5.6.1.

Substance/Preparation

Lemon (Citrus limon) essential oil, organic quality.

Effect

Reduction of body temperature by 0.5 to 1 °C; refreshment and well-being.

Age Suitability

From 3 years onward, the dosage depends on the age of the patient.

Dosage

From 3 years of age: 1 drop lemon essential oil.
   From 6 years of age: 2 drops essential lemon oil.

Instructions

Add an age-appropriate dosage of essential lemon oil to a cup with 1–2 tbsps. of whole milk (alternatively cream, coffee cream, vegetable cream) and mix well. Add the mixture to 2–3 liters of water, and stir together well. The water temperature should be 1–2 °C below the patient's body temperature.

Starting with the arms and legs, wash the skin with a thoroughly wet washcloth, then move on to the torso. Lightly dab the skin and do not dry. The evaporative process, together with the essential lemon oil, has a cooling effect on the skin.

Frequency
After any rise in fever; the prerequisite is that the patient is uniformly warm over the entire body, including hands and feet. There must be no centralization.

Contraindication
Allergy to lemon oil.

Other Applications (3)
Cool (Moist) Wrapped Compresses for the Calf, see Chap. 5.5.6
  Cool (Moist) Wrapped Compresses for the Wrist, see Chap. 5.5.6
  Lemon Slice Compress—for foot sole see Chap. 5.5.8.

6.5.5 Sore Throat

For example, due to:

- Colds
- Tonsillitis
- Pharyngitis

Application (1)
Farmer's Cheese (Quark) Wrapped Compress (Cool)—for neck, see Chap. 5.5.7.

Substance/Preparation
Farmer's cheese (quark), preferably lean (without additives).

Effect
Cooling, decongestant, analgesic.

Age Suitability
From 3 years.

Instructions
Prepare the wrapped compress with farmer's cheese (quark), as described in Chap. 5.5.7 and apply to the patient's neck. The farmer's cheese (quark) must be room-temperature and not come directly from the refrigerator; if it is too cold, the cooling effect is lost due to increased reactive heating/overheating. If applied in the evening, it can also be left overnight.

Frequency
1–2 times per day.

Contraindications
Neurodermatitis, cow milk allergy.

Note
After the acute phase with severe sore throat and swelling has subsided, the compress can be made with farmer's cheese (quark) warmed to body temperature (36–37 °C), as described in Chap. 5.5.7. In the healing phase, the body-warm compress is often more pleasant than the cool compress.

Application (2)
Mustard Flour FootbBath, see Chap. 5.6.6.

Substance/Preparation
Black mustard flour (Semen Sinapis nigrae pulv.)

Effect
Promotes blood circulation, stimulates the metabolism, draining.

Age Suitability
From 3 years of age, the dosage depends on the age of the patient.

Dosage
From 3 years of age: 1 tsp. black mustard flour to approx. 5 liters of water.
   From 6 years of age: 0.5–1 tbsp black mustard flour to approx. 5 liters of water.
   From 12 years of age: 1–2 tbsp black mustard flour to approx. 5 liters of water.

Instructions
Using an age-appropriate dosage, prepare and perform the footbath as described in Chap. 5.6.6.

Frequency
1 time daily.

Contraindications
Skin lesions in the area of application.
   Mustard flour intolerance/allergy.

Note
The wrapped compress (1) and mustard flour footbath (2) can be combined without overloading the organism.

6.5.6 Cough/Bronchitis

The following application is also recommended in cases of *pneumonia*.

Application (1)
Oil Compress—for the chest, see Chap. 5.5.1.

Substance/Preparation
Lavender fine (Lavandula angustifolia), essential oil, organic quality Base oil (neutral oil): olive, sunflower, canola or almond oil.

Effect
Relaxing for spasmodic cough, soothing, antiseptic, balancing.

Age Suitability
From 1 year onward, the dosage depends on the age of the patient.

Dosage
From 1 year of age: 1–2 drops lavender oil to 1 tbsp base oil.
   From 3 years of age: 2–3 drops lavender oil to 1 tbsp base oil.
   From 6 years of age: 3–4 drops lavender oil to 1 tbsp base oil.
   From 12 years of age: 4–5 drops lavender oil to 1 tbsp base oil.

Instructions
Using an age-appropriate dosage, mix the base oil and lavender essential oil in a sealable glass jar. Mix together by gently turning and shaking the jar (1–2 min.).
   Prepare the compress, as described in Chap. 5.5.1, and apply to the patients' chest.

Frequency
1 time per day, preferably in the evening before sleeping. As there is no evaporative cooling effect, the compress can be left on for a longer period of time, even overnight.

Contraindication
Allergy/intolerance to lavender.

Note
If the patient cannot tolerate lavender or its scent, bergamot mint essential oil (Mentha x citrata) can be used as an alternative.

Application (2)
Chest Compress with Mustard Flour and Olive Oil.

Substances/Preparations
Black mustard flour (Semen Sinapis nigrae pulv.)
   Olive oil (base oil).

Effect

Expectorant, respiratory deepening, mildly warming.

This compress is especially suitable for children with sensitive skin and/or cognitive disorders.

Age Suitability

From 1 year onward, the dosage depends on the age of the patient.

Dosage

From 1 year of age: 1 tsp–1 tbsp mustard flour to 1 tbsp olive oil.

From 6 years of age: 2 tbsp mustard flour to 2 tbsp. Olive oil.

From 12 years of age: 3 tbsp mustard flour to 2–3 tbsp. Olive oil.

Preparation and Instructions

Materials

- Black mustard flour.
- Olive oil.
- Small bowl.
- 1 cloth diaper (inner layer)
- 2 Sheets of paper towel or cellulose paper
- 1 Terry cloth washcloth (intermediate layer)
- 1 Molleton fabric or terry cloth towel or, alternatively, a scarf (outer layer) Adhesive tape.

Instructions

In a small bowl, mix (an age-appropriate dosage of) the mustard flour with the olive oil to form a paste. Lay the cloth diaper open and place the paper towel/cellulose paper in the center. Using a knife or spatula, spread the paste over a rectangular area that corresponds with the size of the patient's chest or back. Fold the edges of the diaper toward the center to form a small package.

Place the molleton fabric/terry cloth towel (outer layer) on the patient's bed at their chest level. Fold lengthwise so that its width reaches from the patient's armpits to their ribs (maximum to their waist). Place the compress on their chest or back, so the side of the compress with only one layer of fabric is between the paste and their skin. Cover with the terry cloth washcloth (middle layer).

Wrap the outer layer around the patient so that it fits snugly and the end is secured with adhesive tape. (Caution: because of the risk of injury, do not use safety pins!).

For smaller children, a bodysuit can replace the outer sheet.

Application Time

1–5 years of age: 30 min.

6 years and older: 1 h.

12 years and older: 2 h.

During the first application, check the skin reaction at shorter intervals; *slight* redness may occur. If the patient becomes agitated or if the redness is severe, remove the compress immediately.

Frequency
1 time per day.
Note: redness from previous treatments must have clearly subsided before another application is carried out.

Contraindications
Skin lesions in the area of application,
High fever.
Mustard intolerance/allergy.

Note
Mustard can (mildly) irritate the skin; patients must remain under observation during the entire application. If the irritation is too intense, remove the compress before the end of the recommended treatment time.

Application (3)
Wrapped Ginger Compress, see Chap. 5.5.5.

Substance/Preparation
Ginger powder.

Effect
Warming, respiratory deepening, expectorant.

Age Suitability
From 2 years onward, the dosage depends on the age of the patient.

Dosage
From 2 years of age: 1/2 tsp. ginger powder to 300–400 ml water.
From 6 years of age: 1 tsp. ginger powder to 300–400 ml water.
From 12 years of age: 1 tbsp ginger powder to 300–400 ml water.

Instructions
Prepare and apply as described in Chap. 5.5.5.

Frequency
1 time per day, preferably in the morning or early afternoon before 15:00 h; application later in the day may cause sleep disturbances due to the stimulating effect of ginger. Note: redness from previous treatments must have clearly subsided before the next application is carried out.

Contraindications
Injured skin, acute inflammation and/or sensitivity disorders in the area of application.

Intolerance/allergy to ginger.

Note
If the nipples will have contact with the ginger compress, smear them with petroleum jelly or an oil-based cream without irritants for protection and cover them with gauze or a cotton pad.

Ginger can irritate the skin; patients must remain under observation during the entire application. If the irritation is too intense, stop the treatment before the end of the recommended treatment time.

Application (4)
Warm (Moist) Wrapped Compress—for chest, see Chap. 5.5.2.

Substance/Preparation
Thyme (Thymus vulgaris), tea drug.

Effect
Relief of spasmodic cough, irritable cough and dry cough irritation, warming, anti-inflammatory.

Age Suitability
From 6 years onward, the dosage depends on the age of the patient.

Dosage
From 6 years of age: 1 tsp. of tea drug to 300 ml of water.

From 12 years of age: 1 tbsp tea drug to 300 ml water.

Instructions
Pour 300 ml of boiling water over (an age-appropriate dosage of) the thyme and leave it to infuse for 5 min before straining. Keep the liquid warm (e.g., in a thermos) and do not soak the substance cloth until everything is prepared and the patient is ready for application.

Use this infusion to prepare the compress and apply as described in Chap. 5.5.2.

Place the inner layer (substance cloth) on the front of the chest and cover with a folded terry cloth towel as an intermediate layer. Snugly wrap the outer towel around the chest without folds.

A hot-water bottle with approx. 60 ° C warm water (mix 2/3 boiling hot water with 1/3 cold water) can be placed on the outer wrap to prevent cooling. After 20–25 min., remove the moist inner and middle cloths, before tightly reclosing the outer layer and covering the patient with a warm blanket. During the post-treatment rest period of approx. 30 min, the hot-water bottle can remain in place.

Frequency
1 time daily.

Contraindications
Unstable circulation.
   Intolerance/allergy to thyme.

Application (5)
Mustard Flour Compress—for chest, see Chap. 5.5.3.

Substance/Preparation
Black mustard flour (Semen Sinapis nigrae pulv.)

Effect
Promotes blood circulation, deepens the respiratory tract, releases secretions.

Age Suitability
From 6 years of age.

Dosage
1–2 heaped tbsps of mustard powder—depending on the size of the compress.

Instructions
Prepare and apply as described in Chap. 5.5.3.

Frequency
1 time per day.
   Note: redness from previous treatments must have clearly subsided before another application is carried out.

Contraindications
Sensitive skin, open wounds, acute inflammation and/or sensitivity disorder in the area of application.
   Mustard flour intolerance/allergy.

Note
If the nipples will have contact with the mustard compress, smear them with petroleum jelly or an oil-based cream without irritants for protection and cover them with gauze or a cotton pad.
   Mustard can irritate the skin; patients must remain under observation during the entire application. If the irritation is too intense, stop the treatment immediately to avoid skin burns.
   The mustard compress may also be used in cases of mild fever, to help the body to dissipate heat.

6.5.7   Urinary Tract Infection

The following recommendations also apply to *urinary retention, urinary inconti-nence* and *irritable bladder*.

Application (1)
Mustard Flour Footbath, see Chap. 5.6.6.

Substance/Preparation
Black mustard flour (Semen Sinapis nigrae pulv.)

Effect
Promotes blood circulation, stimulates the metabolism, draining.

Age Suitability
From 3 years onward, the dosage depends on the age of the patient.

Dosage
From 3 years of age: 1 tsp. black mustard flour to approx. 5 liters of water.
   From 6 years of age: 0.5–1 tbsp black mustard flour to approx. 5 liters of water.
   From 12 years of age: 1–2 tbsp black mustard flour to approx. 5 liters of water.

Instructions
Using an age-appropriate dosage, prepare and carry out as described in Chap. 5.6.6.

Frequency
1 time daily.

Contraindications
Skin lesions in the area of application.
   Mustard flour intolerance/allergy.

Note
When there is a tendency to cold feet, the mustard flour footbath can also be used preventively against infections and to improve thermoregulation. In this case, carry out the footbath for 5 days, followed by a 2-day break; this sequence should be repeated for another 2 weeks. If necessary, the treatment series can be repeated after a 3-week break. For additional recommendations, see "Cold Legs and Feet."

Application (2)
Oil Compress—for the bladder area, see Chap. 5.5.1.

Substance/Preparation
Eucalyptus, Oleum aethereum 10%, bath additive; ready-to-use preparation (Wala).

(Although the preparation is called a "bath additive," it can also be used for oil application. It is a mixture of eucalyptus essential oil and olive oil).

Effect
Warming, anti-inflammatory, relaxes the bladder muscles and improves continence.

Age Suitability
From 3 years onward, the dosage depends on the age of the patient.

Dosage
From 3 years of age: 1 tsp. eucalyptus oil 10% diluted with 5 tsp. olive oil (1:5).
From 8 years of age: 1 tsp. eucalyptus oil 10% diluted with 2 tsp. olive oil (1:2).
From 12 years of age: 1 tsp. eucalyptus oil 10% diluted with 1 tsp. olive oil (1:1).
From 15 years of age, eucalyptus oil can be used undiluted.

Instructions
Using an age-appropriate dosage, prepare and apply the compress as is described in Chap. 5.5.1. Place the substance cloth on the lower abdomen, in the area of the bladder.

During application, the feet should be warm or kept warm with a good covering, or if required, with socks (made of natural material such as wool, cotton, silk) or a hot-water bottle (not in cases of sensitivity disorders of legs/feet).

Frequency
1–2 times a day.

Since no evaporative cooling occurs, the compress can be left in place for a longer period of time, for example overnight.

Contraindications
Skin lesions or inflammation in the area of application.

Intolerance/allergy to eucalyptus oil (cineole, main component of eucalyptus oil).

Pseudocroup and bronchial asthma (due to possible hypersensitivity of the respiratory tract).

Application (3)
Sitting Bath, see Chap. 5.6.4.

Substance/Preparation
Tea drugs:

- Sage (Salvia officinalis).
- Thyme (Thymus vulgaris).
- Chamomile (Matricaria chamomilla flos).
- Each to be used separately in a daily rotation.

Effect

Anti-inflammatory, curing (especially sage), antibiotic and antifungal (especially thyme), soothing (especially chamomile), warming, cleansing.

The effect of each substance is meant to complement the effects of the others, use a different substance each day to prepare the sitting bath.

Age Suitability

From 2 years or as soon as the child can sit stably.

Preparation and Instructions

Pour one liter of boiling water over a handful of the corresponding tea drug (in daily rotation), cover and leave to infuse for 5 min. and then strain. Mix this infusion with 5 liters of tap water (mixing ratio 1:5). The bath water temperature should be about 38 °C or a maximum of 2 °C above the patient's body temperature. Fill the sitting tub/washing bowl high enough so that the patient sits in the water up to their navel. (If more bath water is required, prepare more tea infusion to maintain the 1:5 mixing ratio).

Carry out the sitting bath as described in Chap. 5.6.4.

Frequency

1 time daily, in acute situations up to 2 times daily.

Continue the treatment for 5–7 days after the acute symptoms have subsided.

Contraindications

Skin lesions in the area of application. Intolerance/allergy to one or more of the substances.

Note

To support healing and prevent new urinary tract infections, ensure that the patient's feet are kept warm by wearing socks/socks made of natural materials (wool, cotton, silk).

6.5.8 Pneumonia (Pneumonia)

For recommendations, see Cough/Bronchitis.

6.5.9 Middle Ear Infection (Otitis Media)

The following recommendations also apply to **earaches** that occur, for example, in connection with a cold, without the presence of a pronounced middle ear infection.

Application (1)

Onion Ear Bag, see Chap. 5.5.9.

Substance/Preparation
Onion (Allium cepa).

Effect
Analgesic, anti-inflammatory, decongestant.

Age Suitability
From 1 year of age.

Instructions
Prepare and apply the onion ear bag as described in 5.5.9.

Frequency
1–2 times a day.

Contraindications
Skin defects or inflammation in the area of application.

Application (2)
Cotton Ball with Lavender Oil.

Substance/Preparation
Lavender fine (Lavandula angustifolia), essential oil, organic quality base oil (neutral oil): almond, olive or sunflower oil.

Effect
Analgesic, soothing.

Age Suitability
From 1 year of age.

Dosage and Instructions
Put one drop of lavender essential oil on a small cotton ball and carefully place it in the front part of the external auditory canal. Leave in place as long as possible, even overnight.

If the patient cannot tolerate the cotton ball in their ear or having their ear touched, diluted lavender oil (1 drop lavender essential oil with 1 tbsp. Base oil) can be gently massaged behind their ear instead.

Frequency
The lavender oil cotton ball can be replaced up to 2 times a day if necessary.
Rubbing behind the ear, up to 3 times a day.

Contraindication
Allergy/intolerance to lavender.

Note

As an alternative to lavender essential oil, bergamot mint essential oil (Mentha x citrata) can be used in the above dosage.

6.5.10 Pseudocroup, Seizure

Application

Air Humidification with Thyme Infusion.

Substance/Preparation

Thyme (Thymus vulgaris), tea drug.

Materials

Cloth towels, for example, diapers, hand towelsDrying rack, clothesline or other furniture for hanging clothes.

Effect

Relief of cough irritation and spasm.

Age Suitability

All ages.

Preparation and Instructions

Pour 500 ml of boiling water over 1 tsp. of the thyme and leave to infuse for 5 min before straining. In a bowl, dilute this infusion with 1.5 liters of water. Soak several cloth towels in the bowl, wring them out and hang them in the room over a clothes horse, clothesline or radiator so that the moisture can evaporate. As the cloths begin to dry, wet them again.

During a seizure, it may be helpful to sit the patient on your lap and hold his or her feet.

Contraindications

None known.

Notes

Cool room air supports the soothing effect of this application. If the patient does not like the scent of thyme, cloths can also be soaked in plain water.

To avoid additional irritation of the respiratory tract, no other essential oils or fragrant substances should be added to the water.

The thyme infusion stains fabric, this should be taken into account when selecting cloths to use.

6.6   Gastrointestinal Diseases/Disorders

6.6.1   Abdominal Cramps, Colic

The following recommendations also apply to **flatulence** (meteorism).

Application (1)
Oil Compress—for the abdomen, see Chap. 5.5.1.

Substance/Preparation
Melissa oil, ready-to-use preparation (Wala).

Age Suitability
All ages, dosage is based on the age of the patient.

Dosage
0–12 months: Dilute the melissa oil with equal parts (1:1) almond or olive oil, or sunflower oil as a substitute.
    From 1 year of age, the melissa oil can be used undiluted.

Instructions
Prepare and apply as described in Chap. 5.5.1.

Frequency
1–2 times a day if required Since no evaporative cooling occurs, the compress can also be left in place for a longer period, for example overnight.

Contraindications
Unclear abdomen, defective skin in the area of application, inflammatory processes, fever.
    Allergy/intolerance to an ingredient of the preparation, as listed in the instructions for use/content information.

Application (2)
Warm (Moist) Wrapped Compress—for abdomen, see Chap. 5.5.2.

Substance/Preparation
Oxalis essence, ready-to-use preparation (Wala).

Age Suitability
All ages, dosage is based on the age of the patient.

Dosage
0–12 months: ½ tsp. oxalis essence to 250 ml water.
    From 1 year of age: 1 tsp. oxalis essence to 250 ml water.
    From 2 years of age: 1 tbsp oxalis essence to 250 ml water.

Instructions

Mix an age-appropriate dosage of the oxalis essence with 250 ml of tempered water (40 °C). Prepare and apply the abdominal compress as described in Chap. 5.5.2. Allow for 15–30 min. Post-treatment rest.

Frequency

1–2 times per day.

Contraindications

Acute abdomen, inflammation or injury of the skin in the treated areaAllergy/intolerance to an ingredient of the preparation, as listed in the instructions for use/content information.

Application (3)

Rhythmic Embrocation:

- Two-Handed Abdominal Embrocation, see Chap. 5.3.8
- Diamond Formation Embrocation, see Chap. 5.3.

Substance/Preparation

Melissa oil, ready-to-use preparation (Wala) or.
    Oxalis, Folium 10%, ointment, ready-to-use preparation (Weleda).

Age Suitability

0–12 months: Dilute melissa oil with equal parts (1:1) of a neutral oil (almond or olive oil, alternatively sunflower oil).
    From 1 year of age: Melissa oil, undiluted; or Oxalis, Folium 10%, ointment.

Instructions

Using an age-appropriate dosage, rub/massage in 2–3 ml of the oil using the method described in Chap. 5.3. Allow for 10–15 min. Post-treatment rest. During the embrocation and following rest period, take extra care to ensure the patient is kept warm.
    The two-handed abdominal embrocation can also be performed with one hand. In this case, apply the oil to the abdomen using 3–5 circular movements in a clockwise direction, starting from the right groin. In the case of tumors or metastases in the abdomen, the embrocation should be particularly gentle.
    If the abdomen is sensitive to touch, a (rhythmic) foot embrocation (see Chap. 5.3.13) with one of the above preparations can be used as an alternative.

Frequency

If necessary, several times a day, not directly following a meal (approx. 30 min. interval).

Contraindications

Acute abdomen, bleeding in the abdominal regionAllergy/intolerance to an ingredient of the preparation, as listed in the instructions for use/content information.

Effect
Applications 1, 2 and 3 have anti-flatulent, cramp-relieving, analgesic and calming effect.

6.6.2 Flatulence (Meteorism)

For recommendations, see Abdominal cramps, colic.

6.6.3 Diarrhea (Diarrhea)

Application (1)
Oil Compress—for abdomen, see Chap. 5.5.1.

Substance/Preparation
Melissa oil, ready-to-use preparation (Wala).

Age Suitability
All ages, dosage is based on the age of the patient.

Dosage
0–12 months: Dilute the melissa oil with equal parts (1:1) almond or olive oil, or sunflower oil as a substitute.
From 1 year of age, the melissa oil can be used undiluted.

Instructions
Using an age appropriate dosage, prepare and apply the abdominal oil compress abdomen as described in Chap. 5.5.1.

Frequency
1–2 times a day as needed.
Since no evaporative cooling occurs, the compress can also be left in place for a longer period, for example overnight.

Contraindications
Acute abdomen, defective skin in the area of application, inflammatory processes, fever.
Allergy/intolerance to an ingredient of the preparation, as listed in the instructions for use/content information.

Application (2)
Rhythmic Embrocation:

• Two-Handed Abdominal Embrocation, see Chap. 5.3.8.

- Diamond Formation Embrocation, see Chap. 5.3.7.

Substance/Preparation
Melissa oil, ready-to-use preparation (Wala) or.
   Oxalis, Folium 10%, ointment, ready-to-use preparation (Weleda).

Age Suitability
0–12 months: Dilute Melissa oil with equal parts (1:1) neutral oil (almond or olive oil, alternatively sunflower oil).
   From 1 year of age: Undiluted Melissa; Oxalis, Folium 10%, ointment can be used.

Instructions
Using an age-appropriate dosage, rub/massage in 2–3 ml of the oil/ointment using the method described in Chap. 5.3. Allow for 10–15 min. Post-treatment rest. During the embrocation and following rest period, take extra care to ensure the patient is kept warm.
   The two-handed abdominal embrocation can also be performed with one hand. In this case, apply the oil to the abdomen using 3–5 circular movements in a clockwise direction, starting from the right groin. In the case of tumors or metastases in the abdomen, the embrocation should be particularly gentle.
   If the abdomen is sensitive to touch, a (rhythmic) foot embrocation (see Chap. 5.3.13) with one of the above preparations can be used as an alternative.

Frequency
If necessary, several times a day, not directly following a meal (approx. 30 min. interval).

Contraindications
Acute abdomen, bleeding in the abdominal region.
   Allergy/intolerance to an ingredient of the preparation, as listed in the instructions for use/content information.

Effect
The applications (1) and (2) have a regulating effect on gastrointestinal tone, calming and analgesic.

Note
Ensure sufficient intake of liquids to compensate for the loss of fluids and minerals.
   If diarrhea lasts longer than 1–2 days, especially in cases with infants and young children, it is essential to consult a doctor as the loss of fluids and minerals can quickly become life-threatening.

6.6.4 Vomiting

For recommendations, see Nausea/vomiting.

6.6.5 Nausea/Vomiting

Application (1)
Oil Compress—for the abdomen, see Chap. 5.5.1.

Substance/Preparation
Melissa oil, ready-to-use preparation (Wala).

Age Suitability
All ages, dosage is based on the age of the patient.

Dosage
0–12 months: Dilute the melissa oil with equal parts (1:1) neutral oil (almond or olive oil, alternatively sunflower oil).

From 1 year of age, the melissa oil can be used undiluted.

Instructions
Using an age-appropriate dosage, prepare and apply the oil compress as described in Chap. 5.5.1.

Frequency
1–2 times a day as needed.

For nausea associated with food odors, apply approx. 30 min. Before eating.

Since no evaporative cooling occurs, the compress can also be left in place for a longer period, for example overnight.

Contraindications
Acute abdomen, defective skin in the area of application, inflammatory processes, fever.

Allergy/intolerance to an ingredient of the preparation, as listed in the instructions for use/content information.

Application (2)
Rhythmic Embrocation:

- One-handed Abdominal Circles for Infants, see Chap. 5.4.5.
- Two-Handed Abdominal Embrocation, see Chap. 5.3.8.
- Diamond Formation Embrocation, see Chap. 5.3.7.

Substance/Preparation
Melissa oil, ready-to-use preparation (Wala).

Age Suitability
All ages, dosage is based on the age of the patient.

Dosage
0–12 months: Dilute the melissa oil with equal parts (1:1) neutral oil (almond or olive oil, alternatively sunflower oil).

From 1 year of age, the melissa oil can be used undiluted.

Instructions
Using an age-appropriate dosage, rub/massage in 2–3 ml of the oil using the method described in Chap. 5.3. Allow for 10–15 min. post-treatment rest. During the embrocation and following rest period, take extra care to ensure the patient is kept warm.

The two-handed abdominal embrocation can also be performed with one hand. In this case, apply the oil to the abdomen using 3–5 circular movements in a clockwise direction, starting from the right groin. In the case of tumors or metastases in the abdomen, the embrocation should be particularly gentle.

If the abdomen is sensitive to touch, a (rhythmic) foot embrocation (see Chap. 5.3.13) with one of the above preparations can be used as an alternative.

Frequency
1–2 times a day if required, not directly following a meal (approx. 30 min. interval).

Contraindications
Unclear abdomen, appendicitis, intestinal obstruction, bleeding in the abdominal regionAllergy/intolerance to an ingredient of the preparation, as listed in the instructions for use/content information.

Effect
Applications (1) and (2) have calming and cramp relieving effect, supports liver function.

Application (3)
Scent Swab.

Substance/Preparation
Lemon (Citrus limon) essential oil, organic quality.

Effect
Refreshing, nausea relieving.

Age Suitability
From 1 year of age.

Dosage and Application
1–2 drops of the essential oil are dripped onto a cellulose swab or a (paper) hand-kerchief for the patient to sniff.

Frequency
As needed.

Contraindications
None known.

Note
Keeping the swab or handkerchief in a sealable container or plastic bag between uses, helps the scent of the essential oil last longer.

6.6.6 Constipation (Obstipation)

Application (1)
Rhythmic Embrocation:

- Two-Handed Abdominal Embrocation, see Chap. 5.3.8.
- Diamond Formation Embrocation, see Chap. 5.3.7.
- Melissa oil, ready-to-use preparation (Wala).

Age Suitability
All ages, dosage is based on the age of the patient.

Dosage
0–12 months: Dilute the melissa oil with equal parts (1:1) neutral oil (almond or olive oil, alternatively sunflower oil).
   From 1 year of age, the melissa oil can be used undiluted.

Instructions
Using an age-appropriate dosage, rub/massage in 2–3 ml of the oil using the method described in Chap. 5.3. Allow for 10–15 min. Post-treatment rest. During the embrocation and following rest period, take extra care to ensure the patient is kept warm.
   The two-handed abdominal embrocation can also be performed with one hand. In this case, apply the oil to the abdomen using 3–5 circular movements in a clock-wise direction, starting from the right groin. In the case of tumors or metastases in the abdomen, the embrocation should be particularly gentle.
   If the abdomen is sensitive to touch, a (rhythmic) foot embrocation (see Chap. 5.3.13) with one of the above preparations can be used as an alternative.

Frequency
If necessary, several times a day, not directly following a meal (approx. 30 min. interval).

Contraindications
Acute abdomen, appendicitis, intestinal obstruction, bleeding in the abdominal region.

Allergy/intolerance to an ingredient of the preparation, as listed in the instructions for use/content information.

Application (2)
Oil Compress—for the abdomen, see Chap. 5.5.1.

Substance/Preparation
Melissa oil, ready-to-use preparation (Wala).

Age Suitability
All ages, dosage is based on the age of the patient.

Dosage
0–12 months: Dilute the melissa oil with equal parts (1:1) neutral oil (almond or olive oil, alternatively sunflower oil).

From 1 year of age, the melissa oil can be used undiluted.

Instructions
Using an age-appropriate dosage, prepare and apply the oil compress as described in Chap. 5.5.1.

Frequency
1–2 times a day as needed.

Since no evaporative cooling occurs, the compress can also be left in place for a longer period, for example overnight.

Contraindications
Acute abdomen, skin defects in the area of application, inflammatory processes, fever allergy/intolerance to an ingredient of the preparation, as listed in the instructions for use/content information.

Effect
The applications (1) and (2) have a gastrointestinal tone-regulating effect, stimulate the metabolism and promote excretion.

Note
If there is a tendency to constipation, care should be taken to ensure regular and adequate fluid intake.

6.7 Skin Problems and Care

6.7.1 Pressure Ulcer Prevention

Application

Rhythmic Embrocation
Good Night Figure Eights, see Chap. 5.3.6.

Substance/Preparation
Calendula wound ointment, ready-to-use preparation (Weleda).

Effect
Anti-inflammatory, granulation-promoting, disinfectant.

Age Suitability
From 3 months of age.

Instructions
Thinly apply the ointment to the skin where there is risk of pressure ulcers forming and massaged in gently. In the sacrum area, the Goodnight Figure Eights works very well.

Frequency
3 times a day or at each repositioning or at each diaper change.

Contraindications
Intolerance/allergy to an ingredient of the ointment according to the instructions for use.

Note
The ointment can also be used for an already existing grade 1 pressure ulcer.
    Clean the skin with lukewarm water or olive oil using a soft cloth/rag or a (non-sterile) compress.

6.7.2 Eczema

For recommendations, see Itching.

6.7.3 Itching

For example, due to:

- allergies,
- eczema, neurodermatitis, cradle cap,

- dry skin,
- morphine administration,
- chemotherapy,
- liver or kidney diseases,
- psoriasis,
- insect bites.

Application (1)
Therapeutic Whole-Body Wash, see Chap. 5.6.1.

Substance/Preparation
Alkaline salt, ready-to-use preparation.

Effect
Relief of itching, soothing.

Age Suitability
From 1 year of age, the dosage depends on the age of the patient.

Dosage
1–5 years: ½ tsp. alkaline salt to 2 liters of water.
From 6 years of age: 1 tsp. of alkaline salt to 2 liters of water.

Instructions
Using an age-appropriate dosage, add the alkaline salt to the water and mix well. The water should be body-temperature, approx. 35–37 °C, avoid using water that is too cool or too warm. Intense temperature stimulation can increase itching.

The soothing whole-body wash should begin with washing the torso and move toward the extremities, moving in the same direction of hair growth.

Frequency
1–2 times daily,
Depending on the severity of the itching; areas can also be rubbed with a washcloth soaked in the cooled alkaline water or the washcloth can be applied as a cooling compress.

Contraindications
Allergy/intolerance to an ingredient of the preparation, as listed in the instructions for use/content information.

Application (2)
Therapeutic Whole-Body Wash, see Chap. 5.6.1.

Substance/Preparation
Pansy (Viola tricolor), tea drug.

Effect
Relief of itching, soothing.

Age Suitability
All ages, dosage is based on the age of the patient.

Dosage
0–1 year: ½–1 tbsp tea drug.
  From 1 year of age: 1–2 tbsp tea drug.
  From 6 years of age: 2–3 tbsp tea drug.
  From 12 years of age: 3 tbsp tea drug.

Instructions
Pour 500 ml of boiling water over an age-appropriate dosage of the pansy and leave to infuse 5–10 min. Before straining. Mix this infusion with 2–3 liters of cold water in a wash bowl so that the wash water is *body-temperature* (approx. 35–37 °C). Avoid using water that is too cool or too warm as intense temperature stimulation can increase itching.

The soothing whole-body wash should begin with washing the torso and move toward the extremities, moving in the same direction of hair growth.

Frequency
1–2 times a day.

Depending on the severity of the itching; areas can also be rubbed with a washcloth soaked in the cooled pansy water or the washcloth can be applied as a cooling compress.

Contraindication
Allergy/intolerance to pansy.

Other Applications (3)
Farmer's Cheese (Quark) Compress—for localized itching, e.g., after insect bite, see Chap. 5.5.7.

6.7.4   Lip Care

For dry lips and torn corners of the mouth (rhagades), due to:chemotherapychronic wasting diseases vitamin or iron deficiency.

Substance/Preparation
Shea butter pure or as a ready-to-use preparation (lip balm, lip balm stick) with shea butter from various natural cosmetics manufacturers (e.g., Dr. Hauschka, Wala).

Effect
Moisturizing, refattening, anti-inflammatory, skin-regenerating.

Age Suitability
All ages.

Instructions
Apply a thin layer of the shea butter or lip care preparation to the lips up to the corners of the mouth and gently massaged in.

Frequency
Several times a day if needed, last in the evening before going to bed.

Contraindications
None known.

6.8   Oncology

6.8.1   Chemotherapy Side Effects

Loss of appetite, impaired taste, fatigue.

Application (1)
Oil Compress—for the abdomen, see Chap. 5.5.1.

Substance/Preparation
Melissa oil, ready-to-use preparation (Wala)Solum oil, ready-to-use preparation (Wala).

Effect
Symptom relief through stimulation of liver function.

Age Suitability
All ages, dosage is based on the age of the patient.

Dosage
0–12 months: Dilute the selected oil with equal parts (1:1) neutral oil (almond or
olive oil).
    From 1 year of age, any of the oils can be used undiluted.

Instructions
Using an age-appropriate dosage, prepare and apply the oil compress as described
in Chap. 5.5.1. Place the substance cloth in the area of the liver, on the right upper
abdomen and lower ribs.

Frequency

1 time per day, preferably after lunch with approx. 30 min. Interval to the meal.

Since no evaporative cooling occurs, the compress can also be left in place for a longer period, for example overnight.

Contraindications

Acute abdomen, skin defects in the area of application, inflammatory processes, fever.

Allergy/intolerance to an ingredient of the preparation, as listed in the instructions for use/content information.

Note

Applications can be used during the chemotherapy cycle or between cycles.

Other Applications (2)

For recommendations in case of nausea, see Nausea/Vomiting For recommendations in case of exhaustion, see Exhaustion/Exhaustive States.

6.8.2 Metastatic Pain

Application (1)

Oil Compress—for the pain area, see Chap. 5.5.1.

Substance/Preparation

Aconite pain oil, ready-to-use preparation (Wala), especially for bright, shooting pain or.

Solum oil, ready-to-use preparation (Wala), especially for dull pain.

Age Suitability

From 1 year of age: Solum oil.

From 6 years of age: Aconite pain oil.

Instructions

Prepare the compress with the selected oil (note age suitability) and apply to the affected area as described in Chap. 5.5.1.

If the compress is applied to the torso, use a towel or scarf to wrap it. If the compress is applied to the extremities, a large outer towel is not required.

Frequency

1–2 times a day.

Since no evaporative cooling occurs, the compress can also be left in place for a longer period, for example, overnight.

Contraindications

Skin defects in the area of application.

Intolerance/allergy to an ingredient of the preparation used according to the instructions for use/content information.

Note
Aconite pain oil is highly potent and should be dosed carefully.

Application (2)
(Rhythmic) Embrocation:

- Back Embrocation, see Chap. 5.3.6 and.
- Two-Handed Abdominal Embrocation, see Chap. 5.3.8, and
- Foot Embrocation, see Chap. 5.3.13.

Combine the above embrocations and perform in the order listed.

Substance/Preparation
Aconite pain oil, ready-to-use preparation (Wala), especially for bright, shooting pain or.
    Solum oil, ready-to-use preparation (Wala), especially for dull pain.

Age Suitability
From 1 year of age: Solum oil.
    From 6 years of age: Aconite pain oil.

Instructions
Prepare the compress with the selected oil (note age suitability) and apply to the affected area as described in Chap. 5.3.

Frequency
1–2 times a day.

Contraindications
Skin defects in the area of application Intolerance/allergy to an ingredient of the preparation used according to the instructions for use/content information.

Note
Aconite pain oil is highly potent and should be dosed carefully.

Effect
The applications (1) and (2) have a calming, relaxing, analgesic, enveloping effect.

6.8.3 Mucositis

The applications listed below are recommended for the treatment of mucositis with the corresponding symptoms (inflammation of the oral mucosa with ulceration, pain, infection).

Applications for mucositis prophylaxis are described under the indication "Oral care in the course of chemotherapy (mucositis prophylaxis)."

Application (1)
Oral Rinse with Propolis Tincture.

Substance/Preparation
Propolis tincture, 20%, ready-to-use preparation.

Effect
Promotes wound healing, analgesic, antibacterial, antifungal, antiviral.

Age Suitability
From 10 years of age.

Instructions
Add 2–5 drops of tincture to 50 ml of lukewarm water, mix well and have the patients rinse their mouth intensively for 3–5 min. Afterwards, they can either swallow or spit it out.

Frequency
3–5 times a day: after every meal and additionally once between meals.

Contraindications
Allergy to propolis, allergy to bee venoms (allergic skin reactions are rare; interactions with other agents are not known).

Note
An oral rinse with chamomile sage tea as described under "Oral care during the course of chemotherapy," can also be used.

Application (2)
Oral Rinse with Sea Buckthorn Pulp Oil.

Substance/Preparation
Sea buckthorn pulp oil (Hippophae rhamnoides fruit oil), ready-to-use preparation.

Effect
Anti-inflammatory, analgesic, promotes wound healing.

Age Suitability
From 1 year of age, the dosage depends on the age of the patient.

Dosage
From 1 year of age: 1–2 drops sea buckthorn pulp oil.
    From 3 years of age: 2–3 drops sea buckthorn pulp oil.

From 6 years of age: 3–4 drops sea buckthorn pulp oil.
From 12 years of age: 4–5 drops sea buckthorn pulp oil.

Instructions
Use a teaspoon to administer (an age-appropriate dosage of) the oil pure or mixed with a little water, to the mouth. Patients should use their tongues to distribute throughout their oral cavity and spit out after about 5 min. The oil (containing vitamin C) can also be swallowed if there is no fat intolerance.

For young children, use an eyedropper to drizzle oil onto the tongue or a cotton swab to dab onto the oral mucous.

Frequency
3–5 times a day: after every meal and additionally once between meals.

Contraindications
None known.

Note
Sea buckthorn pulp oil does not burn and is well tolerated. Store oil in a cool and dark place, but not in the refrigerator, because it will solidify. Shelf life is up to 1 year.

Protect textiles and delicate surfaces when using because the oil can cause *stains*.

In addition to rinsing with sea buckthorn pulp oil, the mouth can also be rinsed with chamomile sage tea as described under "Oral care during the course of chemotherapy."

Other Applications (3)
For application recommendations for dry lips and/or torn corners of the mouth (rhagades), see Lip care.

6.8.4 Oral Care in the Course of Chemotherapy (Mucositis Prophylaxis)

The recommendations listed below are for mucosal care in normal to slightly altered oral mucosa (dry, pale mucosa and tongue, furrow formation, small ulcerations) for mucositis and infection prophylaxis.

Applications in existing mucositis are described under the indication "Mucositis."

Application (1)
Oral Rinse with Chamomile Tea.

Substance/Preparation
Chamomile (Matricaria chamomilla), tea drug.

Effect
Anti-inflammatory, granulation-promoting, mild analgesic, antibacterial.

Age Suitability
All ages, dosage is based on the age of the patient.

Dosage
0–1 year: 1/2 tsp. tea drug to 250 ml water.
   From 1 year of age: 1 tsp. of tea drug to 250 ml of water.
   From 11 years of age: 1 tsp. of tea drug to 150 ml of water.

Preparation and Instructions
Pour boiling water over (an age-appropriate dosage of) chamomile tea drug and leave to infuse for 2–3 min before straining.
   Rinse the mouth intensively with the lukewarm tea and then spit out. Repeat several times for 3–5 min.
   For infants and young children, carefully dab the entire mouth area with a cotton swab or gauze swab soaked in tea.

Frequency
3–5 times a day; after every meal and before going to bed.

Contraindications
Allergy/Intolerance of chamomile.

Note
Chamomile is suitable for use in infants for mucositis prophylaxis and for mild inflammation and ulceration of the oral mucosa. Do not infuse the chamomile longer than 3 min. Longer infusion time will have a tanning and drying effect, which is not desirable in this application.

Application (2)
Oral Rinse with Sage and Chamomile Tea.

Substance/Preparation
Sage (Salviae officinalis folium), tea drug and chamomile (Matricaria chamomilla), tea drug.

Effect
Anti-inflammatory, antifungal, antibacterial, relieves excessive salivation, tanning.
   The mixture combines the anti-inflammatory and antibacterial action of chamomile with the antifungal action of sage.

Age Suitability
From 1 year onward, the dosage depends on the age of the patient.

Dosage
From 1 year of age: 1/2 tsp. tea drug sage and 1/2 tsp. tea drug chamomile to 250 ml water.

From 10 years of age: 1/2 tsp. tea drug sage and 1/2 tsp. tea drug chamomile to 150 ml water.

Preparation and Instructions
Pour boiling water over (an age-appropriate dosage of) tea drug and leave to infuse for 2–3 min before straining.

Rinse the mouth intensively with the lukewarm tea and then spit out. Repeat several times for 3–5 min.

For infants and young children, carefully dab the entire mouth area with a cotton swab or gauze swab soaked in tea.

Frequency
3–5 times a day; after each meal and before going to bed.

Contraindications
Allergy/intolerance to sage and/or chamomile.

Application (3)
Oral Rinse with Oil/Oil Pulling.

Substance/Preparation
Base oil (neutral oil): almond, sesame or sunflower oil.

Effect
Anti-inflammatory, stimulates the flow of saliva.

Age Suitability
From about 6 years of age, or as soon as the child is able to keep the oil in the mouth for a longer time without swallowing it.

Dosage and Instructions
Spread about 1 tsp. of the oil throughout the mouth, swish for 5–10 min, then spit out; if necessary, rinse briefly with lukewarm water.

Frequency
3–5 times a day; after every meal and before going to bed.

Contraindications
None known.

Note
Choose the oil based on the patient's preference. Almond oil has the most neutral taste and is therefore recommended in cases of taste sensitivity or aversion to the other oils.

Other Applications (4)
For recommendations in cases of pronounced dry mouth, see Dry mouth during chemotherapy. Recommendations for dry lips, torn corners of the mouth (rhagades), see Lip care.

6.8.5 Dry Mouth During Chemotherapy

Application
Oral Rinse with Lemon Oil Mixture/Oil pulling.

Substance/Preparation
Lemon (Citrus limon), essential oil, organic qualityBase oil (neutral oil): almond, sesame or sunflower oil.

Effect
Stimulation of saliva formation, improved moistening of the oral mucosa.

Age Suitability
From about 6 years or as soon as the child is able to keep the oil in the mouth for a longer period of time without swallowing it.The dosage depends on the age of the patient.

Dosage
From 6 years of age: 4 drops lemon oil to 50 ml base oil.
    From 12 years of age: 8 drops lemon oil to 50 ml base oil.

Preparation and Instructions
Combine an age-appropriate dosage of the base oil and lemon essential oil in a sealable glass jar. Mix by gently turning and shaking the jar (1–2 min).
    Spread about 1 tsp. of the oil throughout the mouth, swish for 5–10 min, then spit out; if necessary, rinse briefly with lukewarm water.

Frequency
3–5 times a day; after every meal and before going to bed.

Contraindications
None known.

Note
Choose the oil based on the patient's preference. Almond oil has the most neutral taste and is therefore recommended in cases of taste sensitivity or aversion to the other oils.Store the oil mixture in a cool and dark place, not in the refrigerator. The shelf life is 3 months.

Other Application (2)
Recommendations for dry lips, torn corners of the mouth (rhagades), see Lip care.

6.8.6 Radiation Catarrh/Effects of Radiation

For the possible consequences of radiation therapy, such as *weakness, lack of drive, exhaustion, nausea*, application suggestions can be found in the table of contents under the terms mentioned, and also under "convalescence phase."

6.9 Mental Stress

6.9.1 Fear/Anxiety

For example, before examinations, interventions/surgeries in palliative care.

Application (1)
Therapeutic Whole Body Wash, see Chap. 5.6.1.

Substance/Preparation
Lavender fine (Lavandula angustifolia), essential oil, organic quality.

Effect
Calming, balancing, harmonizing.

Age Suitability
From 1 year of age, the dosage depends on the age of the patient.

Dosage
From 1 year of age: 1–2 drops lavender oil.
  From 4 years of age: 2–3 drops lavender oil.
  From 8 years of age: 3–4 drops lavender oil.
  From 12 years of age: 4–5 drops lavender oil.

Preparation and Instructions
Emulsify (an age-appropriate dosage of) lavender essential oil with 1–2 tablespoons of whole milk (alternatively cream, coffee cream, vegetable cream). Add preparation to 2–3 liters of warm water and mix well.The water temperature should be 38–40 °C, so that during the wash, the patient feels pleasantly warm, despite the evaporative cooling effect on the skin.

This application should be implemented as a soothing wash, as described in Chap. 5.6.1, from the center of the body to the periphery and in the direction of hair growth.

Contraindication
Intolerance/allergy to lavender.

Notes

If the patient does not like the scent of lavender, bergamot mint essential oil (Mentha x citrata) can be used as an alternative. Unlike other types of mint, it does not contain menthol and is therefore suitable for children under 6 years of age. The dosage of the bergamot mint oil corresponds to the dosage of lavender oil.

The bath milk "Lavender Relaxing Bath" (Weleda) can be used instead of the essential lavender oil at the following dosage: 1–12 years of age: ½ bottle-cap Lavender Relaxing Bath to 2–3 liters of water; from 12 years of age: 1 bottle-cap lavender relaxing bath to 2–3 liters of water.

Application (2)

Rhythmic Embrocation:

- Back Embrocation, see Chap. 5.3.6.
- Single-Handed Calf Embrocation, see Chap. 5.3.12.
- Foot Embrocation, see Chap. 5.3.13.

Each embrocation can be performed alone or in combination with the others. When combined, patients should be worked on from their center outward toward their periphery.

The combination of calf and foot embrocations is conceptually intended to have a particularly harmonizing and calming effect on the heart.

Substance/Preparation

Lavender Relaxing Care Oil, ready-to-use preparation (Weleda) or Solum Oil, ready-to-use preparation (Wala).

Age Suitability

From 1 year of age.

Instructions

Rub/massage in 2–3 ml of the selected oil using the method described in Chap. 5.2 Allow for 20–30 min. Post-treatment rest. During the embrocation and following rest period, take extra care to ensure the patient is kept warm.

Frequency

1–2 times a day if required.

Contraindications

Allergy/intolerance to an ingredient of the preparation, as listed in the instructions for use/content information.

Application (3)

Oil Compress—for chest or abdomen, see Chap. 5.5.1.

Substance/Preparation
Lavender Relaxing Care Oil, ready-to-use preparation (Weleda) orSolum Oil, ready-to-use preparation (Wala).

Age Suitability
From 1 year of age.

Instructions
Prepare and apply one of the oil compresses mentioned above, to the chest or abdomen/upper abdomen, as described in Chap. 5.5.1.

If the oil is applied to the abdomen, it should be applied to the upper abdomen at the level of the solar plexus.

Frequency
1–2 times a day if requiredSince no evaporative cooling occurs, the compress can also be left in place for a longer period, for example overnight.

Contraindications
Allergy/intolerance to an ingredient of the preparation, as listed in the instructions for use/content information.

Effect
The applications (2) and (3) have a relaxing, calming, harmonizing and warming effect.

Listlessness
For application recommendations, see Exhaustion/exhaustive states.

6.9.2 Sleep Disorders

Difficulty falling asleep.
  Disrupted sleep.
  Inability to sleep through.

Application (1)
Therapeutic Whole Body Wash, see Chap. 5.6.1.

Substance/Preparation
Lavender fine (Lavandula angustifolia), essential oil, organic quality.

Effect
Calming, balancing, harmonizing.

Age Suitability
From 1 year of age, the dosage depends on the age of the patient.

Dosage

From 1 year of age: 1–2 drops lavender oil.
From 4 years of age: 2–3 drops lavender oil.
From 8 years of age: 3–4 drops lavender oil.
From 12 years of age: 4–5 drops lavender oil.

Instructions

Emulsify (an age-appropriate dosage of) lavender essential oil with 1–2 tablespoons of whole milk (alternatively cream, coffee cream, vegetable cream). Add preparation to 2–3 liters of warm water and mix well. The water temperature should be 38–40 °C, so that during the wash, the patient feels pleasantly warm, despite the evaporative cooling effect on the skin.

This application should be implemented as a soothing wash, as described in Chap. 5.6.1, i.e., from the center of the body to the periphery and in the direction of hair growth.

Contraindication

Allergy/intolerance to lavender.

Note

If the patient does not like the scent of lavender, bergamot mint essential oil (Mentha x citrata) can be used as an alternative. Unlike other types of mint, it does not contain menthol and is therefore suitable for children under 6 years of age. The dosage of the bergamot mint oil corresponds to the dosage of lavender oil.

Application (2)

Footbath, see Chap. 5.6.5.

Substance/Preparation

Lavender fine (Lavandula angustifolia), essential oil, organic quality.

Effect

Calming, balancing, harmonizing.

Age Suitability

From 2 years or as soon as the child can sit stably; dosage depends on the age of the patient.

Dosage

From 2 years of age: 1–2 drops lavender oil.
From 4 years of age: 2–3 drops lavender oil.
From 8 years of age: 3 drops lavender oil.
From 12 years of age: 4 drops lavender oil.

Preparation and Instructions
Emulsify (an age-appropriate dosage of) lavender essential oil with 1–2 tablespoons of whole milk (alternatively cream, coffee cream, vegetable cream). Add preparation to the footbath water and mix well. The water temperature should be no more than 1–2 °C above the patient's body temperature and the water should reach above the ankles.

The footbath is performed in the evening at bedtime, as described in Chap. 5.6.5. Following the footbath, the feet should be kept warm with socks/stockings made of natural materials (wool, cotton, silk).

Contraindications
Skin lesions in the area of application.
Allergy/intolerance to lavender.

Note
If the patient does not like the scent of lavender, bergamot mint essential oil (Mentha x citrata) can be used as an alternative. Unlike other types of mint, this does not contain menthol and is therefore suitable for children under 6 years of age.

The dosage corresponds to the dosage of lavender oil.

Application (3)

- Rhythmic Embrocation:
- Back Embrocation partial or whole, see Chap. 5.3.6.
- Foot Embrocation, see Chap. 5.3.13, or
- Figure Eight Embrocation, see Chap. 5.3.14.

The back and foot embrocations can be used individually or in combination. If combined, first work on the back and then on the feet (from center of the body toward the periphery).

Substance/Preparation
Lavender Relaxing Care Oil, ready-to-use preparation (Weleda) orSolum Oil, ready-to-use preparation (Wala).

Age Suitability
From 1 year of age.

Instructions
At bedtime, rub or massage in 2–3 ml or an amount of the selected oil corresponding to the treated body areas, as described in Chap. 5.3.

Frequency
1–2 times a day if required.

Contraindications

Allergy/intolerance to an ingredient of the preparation, as listed in the instructions for use/content information.

Application (4)

Oil Compress—for Chest or Abdomen, see Chap. 5.5.1.

Substance/Preparation

Lavender Relaxing Care Oil, ready-to-use preparation (Weleda) or.
   Solum Oil, ready-to-use preparation (Wala).

Age Suitability

From 1 year of age.

Instructions

Using one of the oils mentioned above, prepare the oil compress and apply to the chest or abdomen as described in Chap. 5.5.1.

   In the case of abdominal application, place the compress on the upper abdomen at the level of the solar plexus.

Frequency

1 time per day at bedtime.

   Since no evaporative cooling occurs, the compress can also be left in place for a longer period, for example overnight.

Contraindications

Allergy/intolerance to an ingredient of the preparation, as listed in the instructions for use/content information.

Effect

Sleep-promoting and harmonizing, warming and enveloping effect.

6.9.3 Shock, Mental

For example: after accident, injury, great shock or other psychologically stressful situations.

Application (1)

Rhythmic Embrocation:

- Two-Handed Abdominal Embrocation, see Chap. 5.3.8.
- Diamond Formation Embrocation, see Chap. 5.3.7.
- Foot Embrocation, see Chap. 5.3.13.

Each embrocation can be performed alone or in combination with the others. When combined, patients should be worked on from their center outward toward their periphery.

Substance/Preparation
Oxalis, Folium 10%, ointment, ready-to-use preparation (Weleda) for abdominal and diamond formation embrocationSolum oil, ready-to-use preparation (Wala) for foot embrocation.

Effect
Tension relieving, balancing, calming; the foot embrocation also has a "grounding" and stabilizing effect.

Age Suitability
From 1 year of age.

Instructions
Using an age-appropriate dosage, rub/massage in 2–3 ml of the oil (or an amount corresponding to the abdomen) into the abdomen using the method described in Chap. 5.2. Allow for 10–15 min. Post-treatment rest. During the embrocation and following rest period, take extra care to ensure the patient is kept warm.

The two-handed abdominal embrocation can also be performed with one hand. In this case, apply the oil to the abdomen using 3– 5 circular movements in a clockwise direction, starting from the right groin.

During the embrocation of the abdomen, emphasize the upper abdomen (area of the solar plexus), to optimize the positive effect on the autonomic nervous system.

Frequency
1–2 times per day.

Contraindications
Abdominal embrocation: acute abdomenAllergy/intolerance to an ingredient of the preparation, as listed in the instructions for use/content information.

Application (2)
Warm (Moist) Wrapped Compress—for abdomen, see Chap. 5.5.2.

Substance/Preparation
Oxalis essence, ready-to-use preparation (Wala).

Effect
Tension relieving, calming, enveloping, warming.

Age Suitability
All ages, dosage is based on the age of the patient.

Dosage

0–12 months: ½ tsp. oxalis essence to 250 ml water.

From 1 year of age: 1 tsp. oxalis essence to 250 ml water.

From 2 years of age: 1 tbsp oxalis essence to 250 ml water.

Instructions

Mix 250 ml of tempered water (40 °C) with (the age-appropriate dosage of) the oxalis. Prepare and apply the abdominal compress, as described in Chap. 5.5.2, for moist-warm compresses. Cover the area of the solar plexus well with the substance cloth so that the vegetative effect of the compress can be optimized. Allow for 15–30 min. Post-treatment rest.

Frequency

1–2 times per day.

Contraindications

Acute abdomen, inflammation or injury of the skin in the treated areaAllergy/intolerance to an ingredient of the preparation, as listed in the instructions for use/content information.

Note: The wrapped compress for the abdomen works well in combination with the foot embrocation, as described under application (1).

6.9.4 Indifference

Application

Rhythmic Embrocation:

- Back Embrocation, see Chap. 5.3.6.
- Foot Embrocation, see Chap. 5.3.13.

Each embrocation can be performed alone or in combination with the others. When combined, patients should be worked on from their center outward toward their periphery.

Substance/Preparation

Solum oil, ready-to-use preparation (Wala).

Effect

Mood-lifting, harmonizing.

Age Suitability

From 1 year of age.

Instructions
Using an age-appropriate dosage, rub/massage in 2–3 ml of the oil using the method described in Chap. 5.3. Allow for 20–30 min. Post-treatment rest. During the embrocation and following rest period, take extra care to ensure the patient is kept warm.

Frequency
1–2 times a day as required.

Contraindications
Allergy/intolerance to an ingredient of the preparation, as listed in the instructions for use/content information.

6.10   Pain

6.10.1 Headache with Cold

For recommendations, see cold.

6.10.2 Headache, Tension-Related

Application (1)
Rhythmic Embrocation:

- Forehead Embrocation, see Chap. 5.3.3.
- Neck Tension Release, see Chap. 5.3.4.
- Back Embrocation, see Chap. 5.3.6.
- Foot Embrocation, see Chap. 5.3.13.

The embrocations can be applied individually or in combination (sequence: forehead—neck—back—feet).

Substance/Preparation
Aconite Pain Oil, ready-to-use preparation (Wala) orLavender Relaxing Care Oil, ready-to-use preparation (Weleda) orSolum Oil, ready-to-use preparation (Wala).

Effect
Muscle relaxing, draining, analgesic.

Age Suitability
From 1 year of age: Lavender Relaxing Care Oil; Solum Oil.
From 6 years of age: Aconite pain oil (Attention: Do not use for forehead embrocation).

Instructions
Using an age-appropriate dosage, rub/massage in 2–3 ml of the oil (or an amount corresponding to the treatment area) using the method described in Chap. 5.3.

Frequency
1–3 times a day as needed.

Contraindications
Allergy/intolerance to an ingredient of the preparation, as listed in the instructions for use/content information.

Note
Aconite pain oil is highly potent and should be dosed carefully.

Application (2)
Mustard Flour Footbath, see Chap. 5.6.6.

Substance/Preparation
Black mustard flour (Semen Sinapis nigrae pulv.)

Effect
Tension relieving, warming, metabolism stimulating.

Age Suitability
From 3 years onward, the dosage depends on the age of the patient.

Dosage
From 3 years of age: 1 tsp. black mustard flour to approx. 5 liters of water.
    From 6 years of age: 0.5–1 tbsp black mustard flour to approx. 5 liters of water.
    From 12 years of age: 1–2 tbsp black mustard flour to approx. 5 liters of water.

Instructions
Prepare and carry out the footbath as described in Chap. 5.6.6.

Frequency
1 time daily, preferably at symptom onset.
    If there is a tendency for tension-related headaches, the mustard flour footbath can also be used preventively. In this case, the application should be carried out for 5 consecutive days, followed by a break of 2 days; this sequence should be continued for another 2 weeks.
    If necessary, this 3-week treatment series can be repeated after a break of 3 weeks.

Contraindications
Skin lesions in the area of application.
    Allergy/Intolerance of mustard flour.

Application (3)
Footbath with Ginger.

Substance/Preparation
Ginger powder.

Effect
Tension dissipating, lasting warming throughout body.

Age Suitability
From 6 years onward, the dosage depends on the age of the patient.

Dosage
From 6 years of age: 1 heaped tsp. ginger powder to approx. 5 liters of water.
    From 12 years of age: 1 tbsp ginger powder to approx. 5 liters of water.

Preparation and Instructions
In a washing bowl, mix (an age-appropriate dosage of) the ginger with lukewarm water (37–38 °C). The water level should be high enough to reach slightly above the patient's ankles. The patient should wear appropriate clothing and their legs should be covered by a cloth/towel to prevent cooling. The footbath should last 10–20 min. Hot water can be added to the bath in order to maintain the warm temperature, but patients must remove their feet from the bath as the new hot water is being poured in, to prevent burns. Following the footbath, rinse the feet thoroughly, including the area between the toes. Dry well and rub with a care product. A post-treatment rest period of 15–20 min is recommended, but if the patient prefers to move, this is also possible. The feet should be kept warm with socks/socks made of natural materials (wool, cotton, silk).

Frequency
1 time daily, if possible at the onset of symptoms.
    If possible, the application should take place before 15:00 h, application later in the day may cause sleep disturbances due to the stimulating effect of ginger.
    If there is a tendency for tension-related headaches, the ginger footbath can also be used *preventively*. In this case, apply for 5 days, followed by a 2-day break; this sequence should be repeated for another 2 weeks. If necessary, the treatment series can be repeated after a 3-week break.

Contraindications
Skin injuries or diseases, injuries or sensitivity disorders of the feet or lower legs, acute, febrile diseases.
    Intolerance/allergy to ginger.

6.10.3 Muscle Pain (Myalgias)

For recommendations, see musculoskeletal pain.

6.10.4 Neuropathic Pain in Feet/Hands

Application (1)
Footbath, or/and Hand Bath—depending on the localization of the pain—see Chap. 5.6.5.

Substance/Preparation
Alkaline salt, ready-to-use preparation.

Effect
Analgesic, relaxing, soothing.

Age Suitability
From 6 years of age.

Dosage
1 tsp. of alkaline salt with approx. 5 liters of water.

Instructions
In a washbowl, mix the alkaline salt with body temperature water (35–37 °C). Perform the footbath as described in Chap. 5.6.5.

The water level should reach the ankles.

The application time is 10–15 min; except for patients with so-called diabetic feet. In this case, the application should last a maximum of 8 min in order to avoid softening of the skin and the associated increased risk of injury.

During the hand bath, hands should be immersed in water up to the wrists.

The duration of application is 10–15 min.

Frequency
1–time a day, as needed.

Contraindications
Skin injuries in the area of applicationIntolerance/allergy to base salt.

Note
Following the foot or hand bath, an embrocation of the area in pain is recommended, see application (2).

Application (2)
Rhythmic Embrocation, Foot Embrocation see Chap. 5.3.13 and/or
Hand Embrocation, see Chap. 5.3.9.

Substance/Preparation
Aconite pain oil, ready-to-use preparation (Wala).

Effect
Analgesic, relaxing.

Age Suitability
From 6 years of age.

Instructions
Rub/massage 1–3 ml of the oil into the pain area as described in Chap. 5.3.

Frequency
1–2 times, max. 3 times a day if required.

Contraindications
Skin lesions in the area of applicationAllergy/intolerance to an ingredient of the preparation, as listed in the instructions for use/content information.

Note
Aconite pain oil is highly potent and should be dosed carefully.

6.10.5 Earache

For recommendations, see Otitis media.

6.10.6 Back Pain

For recommendations, see Musculoskeletal pain.

6.10.7 Musculoskeletal Pain

On the torso or extremities due to muscular tension (e.g., due to lack of exercise/misalignment)overexertion/cramping (e.g., after exercise).

Application (1)
Rhythmic Embrocation—of the affected area, see Chap. 5.3.

Substance/Preparation
Aconite Pain Oil, ready-to-use preparation (Wala) orArnica Massage Oil, ready-to-use preparation (Weleda) or Hypericum ex herba 5%, Oleum (= St. John's wort oil 5%), ready-to-use preparation (Wala) orSolum oil, ready-to-use preparation (Wala).

Effect
Promotes blood circulation, relaxing, analgesic, warming.

Age Suitability
From 1 year of age: Arnica massage oil, St. John's wort oil (Hypericum ex herba 5%, oleum), Solum oil.
From 6 years of age: Aconite pain oil.

Instructions
Select an age-appropriate oil. Rub/massage 2–3 ml (or a quantity corresponding to the treatment area) into the respective area as described in Chap. 5.3.

Frequency
1–2 times a day.

Contraindications
Skin defects in the area of applicationAllergy/intolerance to an ingredient of the preparation, as listed in the instructions for use/content information.

Note
After the application of St. John's wort oil, do not expose the treated skin to the sun, as there is an increased risk of sunburn.
Aconite pain oil is highly potent and should be dosed carefully.

Application (2)
Oil Compress—in the pain area, see Chap. 5.5.1.

Substance/Preparation
Aconite Pain Oil, ready-to-use preparation (Wala) orArnica Massage Oil, ready-to-use preparation (Weleda) orSolum Oil, ready-to-use preparation (Wala).

Effect
Warming, relaxing, analgesic.

Age Suitability
From 1 year: Arnica massage oil, Solum oil.
From 6 years: Aconite pain oil.

Instructions
Prepare the compress with the selected oil (note age suitability) and apply to the affected area as described in Chap. 5.5.1. If the compress is applied to the extremities, a large outer towel is not required. In the case of application to the torso, a towel or scarf is sufficient for wrapping.

Frequency

1–2 times a daySince no evaporative cooling occurs, the compress can also be left in place for a longer period, for example overnight.

Contraindications

Skin defects in the area of applicationAllergy/intolerance to an ingredient of the preparation, as listed in the instructions for use/content information.

Note

Aconite pain oil is highly potent and should be dosed carefully.

6.10.8 Shoulder Neck Pain

For recommendations, see musculoskeletal pain.

6.11 Injuries

6.11.1 Bruise (Hematoma)

For example, due to:pressure, impact, accident,vascular punctures or other interventionsthrombocytopenia, for example under chemotherapy.

Application (1)

Rhythmic Embrocation—in the hematoma area with "hematoma oil."

Substances/Preparations

Aloe Vera oil, ready-to-use preparationLavender, fine (Lavandula angustifolia), essential oil, organic qualityCistrose/ Cistus (Cistus ladanifer), essential oil, organic qualityImmortelle (Helichrysum italicum), essential oil, organic quality.

Effect

Analgesic, lymphatic drainage stimulating, anti-inflammatory, disinfectant, wound-healing stimulating.

Age Suitability

From 1 year, the dosage depends on the age of the patient.

Dosage

From 1 year of age: 30 ml Aloe Vera oil + 3 drops Lavender oil, fine + 1 drop Cistrose/Cistus oil + 1 drop Immortelle oilFrom 4 years:30 ml Aloe Vera oil + 6 drops Lavender oil, fine + 3 drops Cistrose/Cistus oil + 3 drops Immortelle oilFrom 12 years:30 ml Aloe Vera oil + 10 drops Lavender oil, fine+ + 5 drops Cistrose/Cistus oil + 5 drops Immortelle oil.

In a sealable glass jar, mix the aloe vera oil and (an age appropriate dosage of) essential oils by gently turning and shaking the jar (1–2 min).

Instructions
Gently massage the oil into the skin, using circular motions on the hematoma as well as on the surrounding area so that the tissue is slightly mobilized in the process. In case of open wounds inside the hematoma, use a spatula to thinly coat the wound area with Medihoney 100% (medical honey) and massage the hematoma oil around the wound as described above.

Frequency
In an acute situation, the hematoma oil can be applied hourly, then 2–3 times a day.

Contraindications
Intolerance/allergy to any of the substances used.

Note
The hematoma oil should be stored in a cool and dark place, but not in the refrigerator; it has a shelf life of 3 months.

Application (2)
Compress in the hematoma area.

Substances/Preparation
Immortelle water (immortelle hydrolate), finished preparation.

Effect
Anti-inflammatory, analgesic, promotes lymphatic drainage.

Age Suitability
From 3 years.

Instructions
Use well-chilled Immortelle water from the fridge to soak cotton pads or gauze compresses. Apply to the hematoma and leave for 10–30 min. Depending on the severity of the hematoma, longer if necessary. In case of open wounds inside the hematoma, use a spatula to thinly coat the wound area with Medihoney 100% (medical honey) and apply the soaked compress around the wound.

Frequency
3 times a day.

Contraindication
Allergy/intolerance to Immortelle.

Note

Immortelle water should be stored in the refrigerator so that it is already chilled when needed.

6.11.2 Concussion

Application

Arnica Cap, see Chap. 5.5.10.

Substance/Preparation

Arnica essence, ready-to-use preparation (Weleda; Wala).

Effect

Relief of injury-related symptoms such as headache, dizziness, nausea.

Age Suitability

From 1 year.

Instructions

Prepare and apply the arnica cap as described in Chap. 5.5.10.

Frequency

1–2 times per day

The application should be continued for several days after the acute symptoms have subsided.

Contraindications

Skin injuries in the area of applicationIntolerance/allergy to arnica or other daisy plants (e.g., yarrow).

Note

If the symptoms persist for more than 2–3 days, a doctor should be consulted.

6.11.3 Bruise (Contusion)

The following recommendations also apply to **sprain** and **strain**.

Application (1)

Arnica Compress—for the affected area.

Substance/Preparation

Arnica essence, ready-to-use preparation (Wala; Weleda).

Effect

Analgesic, resorptive, decongestant.

Age Suitability

From 1 year onward, the dosage depends on the age of the patient.

Dosage

1–5 years: 1 tsp. arnica essence to 250 ml water.
   From 6 years of age: 1 tbsp arnica essence to 250 ml water.

Preparation and Instructions

Material: Small wash bowl, substance cloth (thin cloth of cotton, linen) according to the size of the affected area, folded 4 times, outer wrap (terry cloth towel).

   In a wash bowl, mix (an age-appropriate dosage of) the arnica essence with 250 ml of water that is just below body temperature. Dip the inner cloth into this solution, wring out and place on/around the affected body area. Wrap the outer towel around the outside as a moisture barrier. As soon as the inner towel has warmed up, soak it with the arnica solution again and reapply.

Frequency

In acute cases, it is advisable to continue the application for several hours, repeatedly soaking the substance cloth with the arnica solution.

Contraindications

Open skin lesions or sensitive skin in the area of applicationAllergy/intolerance to an ingredient of the preparation, as listed in the instructions for use/content information.

Note

As healing progresses, treatment can be continued with arnica jelly (ready-made preparation from Weleda) first, and then with arnica ointment (ready-made preparation from Wala or Weleda).

Application (2)

Farmer's Cheese (Quark) Compress (cool), see Chap. 5.5.7.

Substance/Preparation

Farmer's cheese (Quark), preferably lean (without additives).

Effect

Cooling, analgesic, decongestant.

Age Suitability

From 1 year of age.

Instructions
Prepare and apply the farmer's cheese (Quark) compress to the affected area as described in Chap. 5.5.7.

Frequency
2–3 times a day.

Contraindications
Neurodermatitis, cow milk allergy.

Note
Particularly with smaller children, ensure that they are dressed or covered during the local cooling application so that they do not generally cool down.

6.11.4 Shock, Mental—After Accident, Injury

For recommendations, see Mental stress > Shock, mental.

6.11.5 Sprain (Distortion)

For recommendations, see Bruise (Contusion).

6.11.6 Strain (Distension)

For recommendations, see Bruise (Contusion).

References

1. Louis, Natalie: Naturopathy for children—colds (script/brochure); 3rd ed., Berlin
2. Scripts written by nurses in the Department of Pediatrics and Adolescent Medicine at Herdecke Community Hospital
3. Scripts and advice from nursing experts for anthroposophic nursing at the Havelhöhe Community Hospital, Berlin
4. Vademecum—External applications in anthroposophic medicine. https://www.pflege-vademecum.de

Substances

7

Clarisse Oberle

7.1 Single Substances

7.1.1 Aloe Vera: *Aloe Barbadensis*

Plant Family Asphodelaceae

Species *aloe vera barbadensis miller*

Origin South America

Composition Anthranoids: aloin A and B, aloinoside A, mucopolysaccharides, flavonoids, saponins, long-chain polysaccharides

Brief Overview of Tradition as a Remedy The aloe plant was used in ancient times. The Egyptian queen Cleopatra was known to care for her skin with aloe extracts, and soldiers wounded during the expansion of Alexander the Great were treated with the plant. Christopher Columbus described the plant as "a doctor in a

C. Oberle (✉)
Charité - Universitätsmedizin Berlin, Berlin, Germany
e-mail: Clarisse.oberle@charite.de

© The Author(s), under exclusive license to Springer Nature
Switzerland AG 2022
G. Seifert, A. Längler (eds.), *The Healing Power of Touch – Guidelines for
Nurses and Practitioners*, https://doi.org/10.1007/978-3-030-85507-9_7

Fig. 7.1 Aloe vera [1]

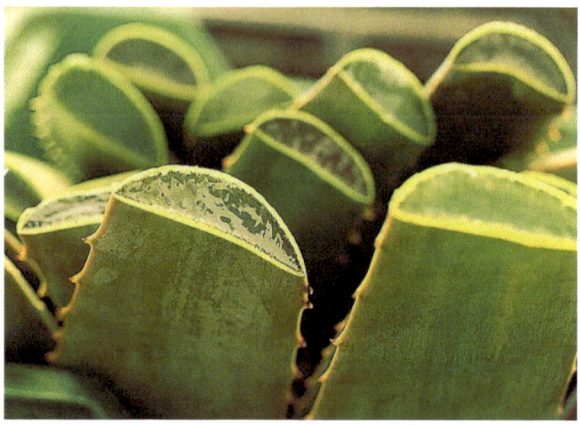

pot." Later, uses expanded for this plant with gel-like substance of the thick-fleshed leaves was used for abdominal cramps, stomach cleansing, and as a laxative (Fig. 7.1).

Effects
– cooling in case of heat conditions, or congestion in tissues
– skin soothing
– anti-inflammatory
– moisturizing
– soothing itching

Range of Use
Internal
– for short-term treatment of constipation, has a laxative effect

External
– For superficial wound care
– For psoriasis and allergic skin reactions
– For tissue congestion
– For sunburn
– For decubitus grade I
– As a prophylaxis against inflammation of the mucous membranes of the mouth
– As an overlay or nipple embrocation for nursing mothers.

External Forms of Application
– As aloe vera oil (e.g., from Primavera) in pure form or as a carrier oil mixed with essential oils, e.g., for hematoma treatment
– As a wound dressing in the form of a gel or fresh juice.

Contraindication Allergy to the ingredients and allergic skin reaction [2, 3]

7.1.2   Arnica Flowers: *Arnicae Flos*

Plant Family   Asteraceae

Species   *arnica montana*

Origin   Europe

Composition   sesquiterpene lactones: Helenalin, dihydro helenalin, flavonoids, essential oil, phenolic carboxylic acid: chlorogenic acid, coumarins.

Brief Overview of Tradition as a Remedy   In the Middle Ages, tinctures from roots and flowers were used for inflammations of all kinds. From the eighteenth century onward, the plant was used for phlebitis, varicose veins, bruises, injuries, gout, and rheumatism, but also as an abortifacient (Fig. 7.2).

Effects
– Anti-inflammatory
– Analgesic
– Antibacterial, antiviral, antifungal.

Range of Use
External (only)
– For treatment of blunt injuries, strains, contusions, and hematomas
– For muscle and joint pain and tension
– For back pain
– For headache
– For gingivitis and aphthae
– For insect bites.

External Forms of Application
– As ointment, gel, tincture, body oil, and mouthwash solution
– As arnica massage oil (e.g., from Weleda) for back embrocation or as an oil application on the painful area
– As arnica essence (e.g., from Wala or Weleda) diluted for poultices according to the package insert.

Contraindication   allergy to the ingredients, in case of injured or irritated skin, open wounds, allergic skin reactions and skin irritations

Note   Do not use on the eye, do not use undiluted [2, 4].

Fig. 7.2 Arnica [1]

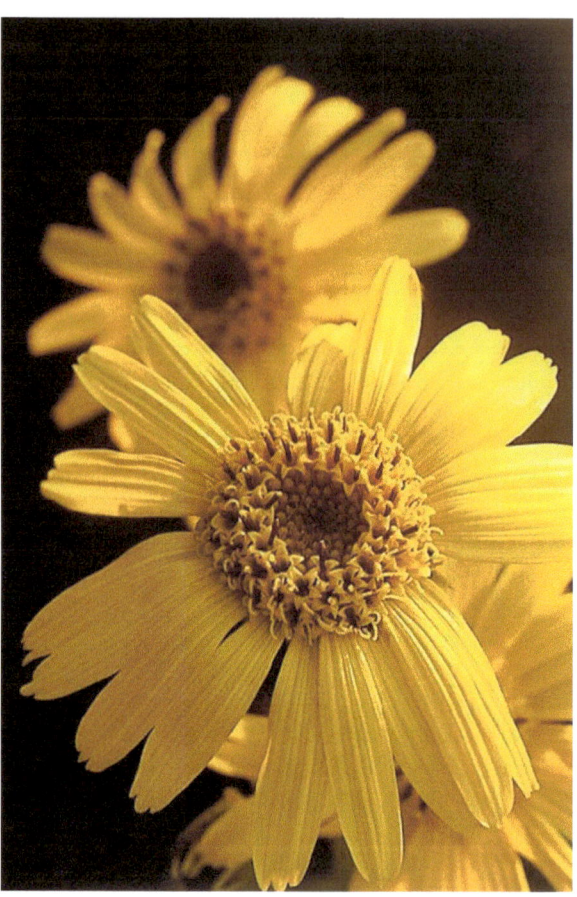

7.1.3   Bee Propolis (Bee Glue): *Propolis*

Origin Propolis is produced when the bees collect resin from hardwood trees and shrubs are enriched with endogenous substances and transformed into a glue.

Composition flavonoids, phenolic carboxylic acid derivatives, hydroxyacetophenone, cinnamaldehyde, chrysin, benzyl alcohols, wax, essential oil, tripertene

Brief Overview of Tradition as a Remedy Propolis has been known since ancient times. In World War II, it was used to treat wounds.

Effects
– Antibacterial, antifungal, antiviral
– Wound-healing
– Anti-inflammatory

– Antioxidant
– Against caries.

Range of Use
External (only)
– For inflammation of the oral mucosa
– For the treatment of skin disease such as cold sores.

External Forms of Application
– Propolis tincture 20% for mouth rinse, e.g., for mucositis
– As mouth rinse for oral care
– In body care products as ointment and cream.

Contraindication Allergy to the ingredients, allergy to bee venom, allergic contact dermatitis [2]

7.1.4 Eucalyptus Leaves: *Eucalypti Folium*

Plant Family Myrtaceae

Species *Eucalyptus radiata*

Origin Australia

Composition 1.2–3% essential oil: 1.8-cineole, monoterpenes: pinene, limonene, pinocarveol, sesquiterpenes.
  Eucalyptus radiata does not contain ketones and is therefore suitable for children and pregnant women.

Brief Overview of Tradition as a Remedy Used in folk medicines since the nineteenth century in Europe, when it was brought to the continent by German-Austrian physician, botanist, and geographer Baron Ferdinand von Müller who learned about eucalyptus from the Aboriginal people of Australia. This was used for colds, asthma, whooping cough, for gastrointestinal complaints, worm diseases, infectious skin diseases, and bladder diseases.

Effects
– Antibacterial
– Expectorant
– Expectorant and cough suppressant
– Freeing the respiratory tract

– Anti-inflammatory
– Stimulates blood circulation
– Diuretic.

Range of Use
Internal
– For colds
– For fever
– For infections of the upper and lower respiratory tract and for support of asthmatic diseases
– For bladder weakness, cystitis, and urinary retention.

External
– For colds, flu-like infections
– For infections of the upper and lower respiratory tract (e.g., sinusitis, acute and chronic bronchitis)
– For local muscle pain, rheumatic complaints
– For inflamed insect bites
– For wounds and burns
– For headaches and concentration difficulties
– For stress-related fatigue.

External Forms of Application
– As a balsam for colds
– As essential oil dissolved in carrier oil (e.g., eucalyptus oil 10%, Wala), e.g., for an oil compress for urinary tract infections
– As bath oil.

Contraindication Allergy to the ingredients and hypersensitivity

Note Concentrated eucalyptus oil is irritating to mucous membranes, it should always be used diluted [2].

7.1.5 Fennel, sweet: *Foeniculi Dulcis Fructus*

Plant Family Apiaceae

Species *foeniculum vulgare*

Origin Mediterranean area

Composition essential oil, anethole, fenchone, estragole, monoterpenes: pinene, limonene

Brief Overview of Tradition as a Remedy Used in Ancient Greece during the times of Hippocrates. The Greek physician Dioscorides used it to increase milk production in nursing mothers, for kidney ailments, and for snake bites. In Europe it has been used since the fifteenth century for gastric distress, digestive weakness, as well as respiratory problems.

Effects
- Antibacterial, antiviral, antifungal
- Decongestant
- Mucolytic
- Expectorant
- Anti-inflammatory

Range of Use
Internal and External
- Relieves cramps in the gastrointestinal tract, e.g., three-month colic in babies, abdominal pain, constipation, and flatulence
- Expectorant—and eases coughs caused by colds.

External Forms of Application
- As carrier oil fennel—caraway (cumin) oil for dissolving essential oils for abdominal rubbing in abdominal cramps, flatulence, and constipation

Contraindication Allergy to the ingredients, allergic reactions in the skin and respiratory tract [2]

7.1.6 Immortelle (Sandy Everlasting): *Helichrysi Flos*

Plant Family Asteraceae

Species *helichrysum arenarium*

Origin Central, Eastern, Southern Europe

Composition flavonoids, essential oil: italidiones and bitter substances

Brief Overview of Tradition as a Remedy Immortelle has a long tradition of medicinal use on the European continent. It was already used in ancient times as a remedy for a wide range of effects. Since the sixteenth century, it was known as a sedative, nervine, and antispasmodic, especially for bilious complaints and as a diuretic.

Effects
- Antibacterial
- Anti-inflammatory
- Wound healing, cell regenerating
- Stimulates blood circulation
- Decongesting and stimulating lymph flow.

Range of Use
External (only)
- For hematomas in wounds
- For sports injuries, contusions, and sprains
- For lymphatic congestion.

External Forms of Application
- As immortelle water (immortelle hydrolate) (e.g., from Primavera) for hematomas, contusions, and sore muscles
- As essential oil dissolved in carrier oil, e.g., for hematomas.

Contraindication Allergy to the ingredients, allergic skin reaction [3]

7.1.7 Ginger Root (Rhizome): *Zingiberis Rhizoma*

Plant Family Zingiberaceae

Species *zingiber officinale*

Origin Southeast Asia, India, China

Composition 1.5–3% essential oil, pungents: gingerols, shogaols

Brief Overview of Tradition as a Remedy Was used medicinally on the Asian continent for thousands of years, known use in Europe is described by the ancient Greek physician Dioscorides as a digestive, and as stimulating and good for the stomach.

Effects
- Stimulates and promotes blood circulation
- Antiemetic
- Antibacterial, antiviral, and antifungal
- Decongestant
- Secretion dissolving
- Analgesic

- Anti-inflammatory
- Digestive and anti-flatulent
- Stimulation of diuresis
- Antioxidant.

Range of Use
Internal
- For nausea and vomiting
- For appetite stimulation in case of loss of appetite
- For the onset of flu and colds
- For mild, cramp-like gastrointestinal complaints
- For motion sickness.

External
- For bronchitis, asthma (not in seizure states), and pneumonia as a compress
- For cold conditions
- For muscle tension and back pain
- For rheumatism and arthritis
- For kidney diseases
- For fatigue.

Forms of Application
Internal
- As tea.

External
- As ginger powder in water as ginger footbath, e.g., for cold feet and cystitis
- As a chest compress, a compress with ginger powder, e.g., for bronchitis and pneumonia.

Contraindication   Allergy to the ingredients, fever, hypertension

Note   Ginger powder is irritating to the skin and may cause a strong sensation of heat [2, 4]

7.1.8   St. John's Wort: *Hyperici Herba*

Plant Family   Hypericaceae

Species   *hypericum perforatum* L.

Origin   Germany, Eastern Europe, and Chile

Composition Hypericins, hyperforins, flavonoids, procyanidins, xanthones, phenolic carboxylic acids, essential oil (sesquiterpenes)

Brief Overview of Tradition as a Remedy Since ancient times, St. John's wort has been used as a medicinal herb, making it one of the oldest medicinal plants in Europe. As a European folk medicine, St. John's wort has long been used as an oil for burns and against nervous disorders and melancholy.

Effects
– Mood enhancing
– Anxiety-relieving
– Balancing
– Stimulates blood circulation
– Anti-inflammatory
– Analgesic.

Range of Use
Internal
– As a dry extract for mild to moderate depression
– For symptoms of stress and mental exhaustion
– To support emotional balance
– For anxiety and restlessness
– For gastrointestinal complaints.

External
– For minor skin inflammations and superficial small wounds
– For anxiety, restlessness, and symptoms of exhaustion
– For muscular pain
– For 1st degree burns (e.g., sunburn).

External Forms of Application
– As an oily liniment (see Chap. 6 Indications) e.g., with Hypericum ex herba 5% (Wala)

Contraindication Allergy to the ingredients

Note When used internally, interactions with other medications may occur causing skin hypersensitivity to sunlight [2, 4].

7.1.9 Chamomile Flowers: *Matricariae Flos*

Plant Family Asteraceae

Species *matricaria recutita*

Origin Southern Europe, Eastern Europe, Southwest Asia

Composition essential oil, flavonoids, coumarin Bisabolol, En-In-Dicycloether, Chamazulene Guaavan derivatives: spathulenol, chamaviolin, Mucilages: fructan, rhamnogalacturonan

Brief Overview of Tradition as a Remedy Chamomile was a very popular medicinal plant dating back to ancient Greece. The ancient Greek physician, Dioscorides, describes it as a remedy for childbirth, flatulence, cystitis, and liver ailments. It has been used since the fifteenth century as a digestive, decongestant, antispasmodic, diuretic, and internal wound-healing element.

Effects
– Antisp asmodic for mild cramp-like complaints in the gastrointestinal tract in three-month colic, abdominal pain, constipation, and flatulence
– Anti-inflammatory
– Wound-healing
– Antibacterial in dermatoses and atopic eczema

Range of Use
Internal
– For cramps and flatulence in the gastrointestinal tract
– For problems with falling asleep and nervousness
– With symptoms of a common cold
– For rhinitis and sinusitis

External
– For inflammations in the mouth and throat area
– For gingivitis
– For inflammations in the anal and genital area
– For minor skin inflammations, superficial wounds, and small boils.

External Forms of Application
– As tea infusion for compresses
– As a mouth rinse for inflammation of the oral mucosa
– As a sitting bath for soreness
– As a wrapped compress, e.g., for flatulence.

Contraindication allergy to the ingredients; do not use on the eye [2, 4, 5]

7.1.10 Caraway: *Carvi Fructus*

Plant Family Apiaceae

Species *carum carvi*

Origin Eurasia

Composition essential oil, carvone, limonene, monoterpenes: pinene, sabinene, myrcene, phellandrene, carene, carveol, flavonoids: camphor oil, quercetin glycosides

Brief Overview of Tradition as a Remedy Caraway has been used for centuries on the European continent as a digestive and purgative, also to increase milk production in nursing mothers, in mouthwash for gargling and for skin-irritating embrocation.

Effects
- Aantispasmodic
- Antibacterial, antiviral, antifungal
- Anti-inflammatory.

Range of Use
Internal
- Decongestant for digestive disorders in the gastrointestinal tract, abdominal pain, flatulence, and constipation

External
- Decongestant for digestive disorders of the gastrointestinal tract in three-month colic, abdominal pain, and constipation
- As a deflating agent for flatulence and bloating.

External Forms of Application
- Dissolved in an oil such as fennel (cumin) caraway oil for children for abdominal embrocation, e.g., for colic.

Contraindication Allergy to the ingredients [2]

7.1.11 Lavender Flowers: *Lavandulae Flos*

Plant Family Lamiaceae

Species *lavandula angustifolia*

Origin Mediterranean area

Composition essential oil, linalyl acetate and linalool, flavonoids, coumarins and tannins

Brief Overview of Tradition as a Remedy Lavender was used by the Egyptians, Romans, and Greeks. Dioscorides described lavender as a remedy, Paracelsus used it as a sedative. Since the sixteenth century in Europe, lavender has been cultivated in monastery gardens and used as a sedative, nervine, and antispasmodic (Fig. 7.3).

Effects
- Soothing
- Antiseptic
- Antispasmodic
- Antianxiety, antidepressant.

Fig. 7.3 Lavender [1]

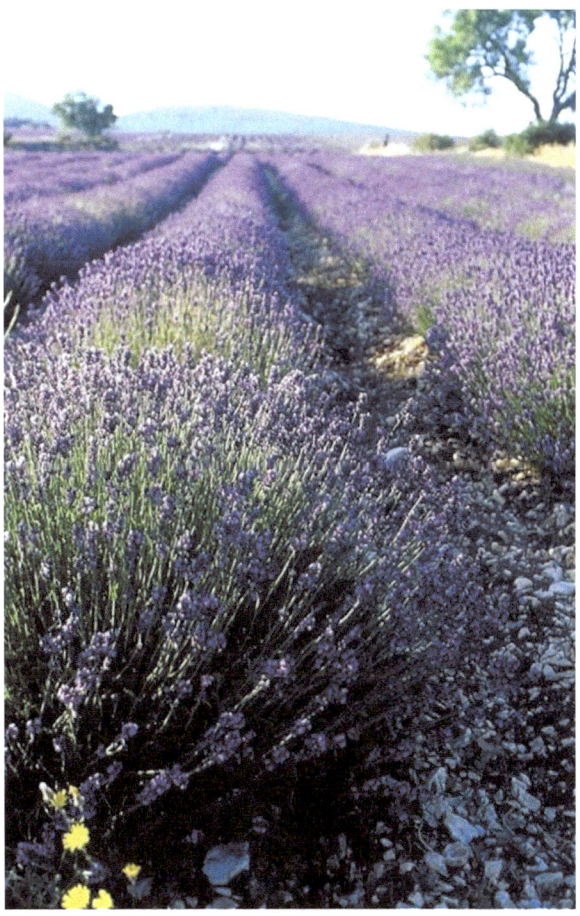

Range of Use
Internal
– For anxiety and restlessness
– For symptoms of stress and exhaustion
– For problems with falling asleep and staying asleep
– For migraines
– For upper abdominal discomfort
– For the treatment of functional circulatory disorders.

External
– For symptoms of stress and exhaustion
– For problems with falling asleep and staying asleep
– For bronchitis.

External Forms of Application
– Essential oil as an additive to bath milk (e.g., from Weleda) for a soothing full body wash
– As essential oil in oil mixtures for embrocation or oil compresses
– Dried flowers in herbal pillows against sleep disorders

Contraindication Allergy to the ingredients, in case of allergic skin reaction [2, 4]

7.1.12 Mallow Flowers: *Malvae Sylvestris Flos*

Plant Family Malvaceae

Species *malva sylvestris*

Origin Europe

Composition mucilages from carbohydrates: galactose, glucuronic acid, galacturonic acid, anthocyanins: malvin, tannins

Brief Overview of Tradition as a Remedy Mallow was used as a remedy in ancient times on the European continent. In Greek and Roman times, the physician Dioscorides recommended drinking mallow juice daily for general well-being. In the fifteenth century, mallow was used for cough and hoarseness, for "rot in the mouth" and for "consumption" (Fig. 7.4).

Effects
– Anti-inflammatory
– Soothing

Fig. 7.4 Mallow [1]

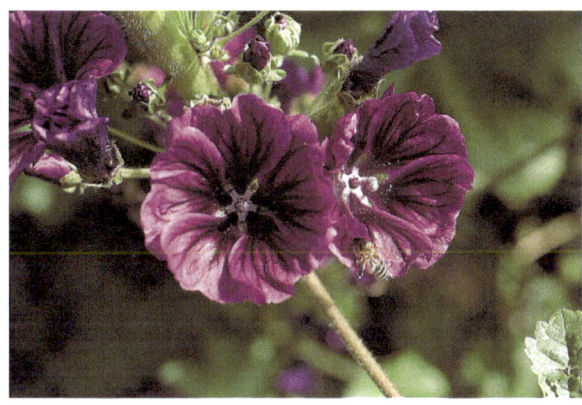

Range of Use
Internal
– Against cough and for flu-like infections
– For inflammations in the mouth and throat area
– For diarrhea and gastritis.

External
– For neurodermatitis and highly sensitive skin
– For irritation of the mucous membrane
– For nervousness and nervous exhaustion
– For insomnia
– For convalescence
– In case of failure to thrive, restlessness, and weakness (infants).

External Forms of Application
– As embrocation with mallow oil (e.g., from Wala) in case of exhaustion, strengthening and calming
– For body care in baby cream (e.g., from Weleda)
– For babies and children with highly sensitive skin.

Contraindication   allergy to the ingredients, in case of hypersensitive reactions [2]

7.1.13 Horseradish: *Armoracia Rusticana*

Plant Family   Brassicaceae

Species   *cochlearia armoracia*

Origin   Europe

Composition   Glucosinolates

Fig. 7.5 Horseradish [1]

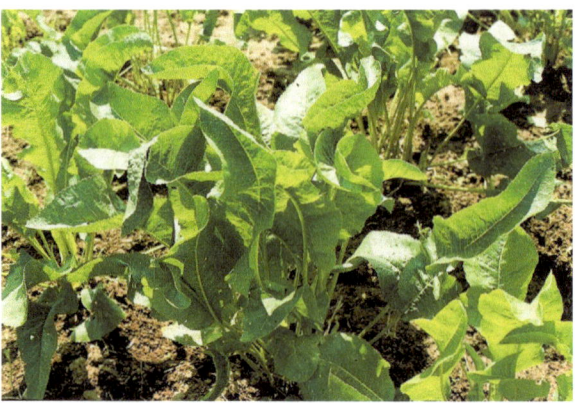

Brief Overview of Tradition as a Remedy   Horseradish root is a household remedy for colds that has been known and used since the European Middle Ages (Fig. 7.5).

Effects
– Antibacterial and antiviral
– Stimulates blood circulation

Range of Use
External (only)
– For catarrh of the upper respiratory tract
– For colds such as rhinitis and sinusitis
– For infections of the urinary tract and urinary retention
– To promote blood circulation in the skin.

External Forms of Application
– As a grated root for compresses.

Contraindication   allergy to the ingredients

Note   Horseradish is irritating to the skin and may cause intense heat and blistering [3, 4, 6].

7.1.14 Melissa Leaves: Melissae *Folium*

Plant Family   Lamiaceae

Species   *melissa officinalis*

Origin   Eastern Mediterranean, Western Asia

Composition Hydroxycinnamic acid derivatives: rosmarinic acid, flavonoids, triterpenes, 1.3-benzodioxol aldehyde, essential oil: citral, geraniol, neral, citronellal, glycosides, tannins

Brief Overview of Tradition as a Remedy Melissa has been used as a medicinal herb since ancient times. Its mood-lifting effect was well known. Melissa was already mentioned by the German Benedictine abbess and healer Hildegard von Bingen. Since the fifteenth century, it has been used variously as a sedative, antispasmodic, digestive and deflating agent, for colds as a diaphoretic, nervine, and invigorating agent, for functional circulatory weakness, nervous palpitations, migraine, hysteria, melancholy, and nervous stomach (Fig. 7.6).

Effects
– Calming, stress-relieving, and anxiety-relieving
– Antiviral and antibacterial
– Antispasmodic
– Sleep-inducing
– Anti-flatulence.

Range of Use
Internal
– For mild stress symptoms and nervous sleep disturbances
– For mild cramp-like gastrointestinal complaints and flatulence
– For colds and flu-like infections with coughing.

External
– For anxiety, restlessness, irritability, and tension
– For states of exhaustion
– As a topical application for cold sores.

Fig. 7.6 Melissa [1]

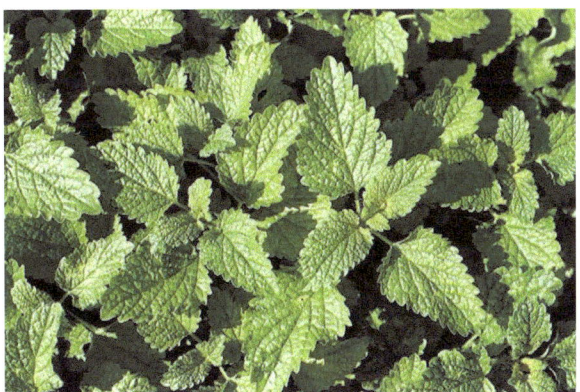

External Forms of Application
- As an embrocation with melissa oil (e.g., from Wala) for anxiety, restlessness, and nervousness; for abdominal cramps, flatulence, constipation, loss of appetite, and vomiting
- As bath oil for relaxation (e.g., Melissa ex herba 5%, Wala) [2, 4].

7.1.15 Peppermint Leaves: *Menthae Piperitae Folium*

Plant Family Lamiaceae

Species *Mentha X Piperita*

Origin Is obtained exclusively from crops in Bavaria, Thuringia, Spain, and Bulgaria

Composition menthol, menthone, cineole, limonene, essential oil: Mentha piperitae aetheroleum, rosmarinic acid, caffeic acid derivatives, flavonoids and triterpenes

Brief Overview of Tradition as a Remedy Mint is one of the oldest medicinal plants already used by the ancient Egyptians, and 2000 years ago, in the Asian region. Dioscorides described mint as being good for the stomach. In Europe, it was first cultivated in England in the seventeenth century and then spread to Central Europe. To this day, peppermint is one of the most widely used medicinal plants.

Effects
- Antispasmodic and relaxing for digestive problems
- Antispasmodic for mild cramp-like complaints in the gastrointestinal tract
- Antibacterial
- Cooling.

Range of Use
Internal
- For digestive problems
- For functional gastrointestinal complaints.

External
- For fever
- For muscular pain
- For tension headache and migraine
- For febrile colds and coughs
- For itching and hives.

External Forms of Application
– As a tea infusion, e.g., for a whole-body wash in case of fever
– As an essential oil dissolved in a carrier oil, e.g., for a neck embrocation for headaches
– As an application to the temple area in case of headache.

Contraindication allergy to the ingredients

Note Concentrated peppermint oil irritates mucous membranes, it should always be used diluted. Do not use on babies, young children up to 6 years, and pregnant women [2, 4].

7.1.16 Farmer's Cheese (Quark): *Massa Lac Bovinae Ferment et Inspiss*

Origin German-speaking Central Europe Soft curd cheese, farmer's cheese, or in German, quark, is a freshly fermented white cheese that has a consistency between yoghurt and cottage cheese and originates from the German and slovic-speaking countries of Central Europe. *Quark* is made by the acidification of milk that separates the curd from the whey; a process that continues in a compress when applied to the skin. As a chosen compress for cooling and pain-relief, *quark* may have varying consistencies in different countries. Here a farmer's cheese made with whole milk that isn't too wet is most suitable to support expectorant and relaxing effects of *quark* [2, 7].

Composition acidum lacticum, lactose

Effects
Due to the whey contained in the cheese, the following effects occur:

– Cooling
– Analgesic
– Anti-inflammatory
– Decongestant.

Range of Use
External (only)
– For hematomas, bruises, and sprains
– For itching
– For insect bites and sunburn
– For moist rattling breathing, bronchitis, and pneumonia
– For headaches
– For bursitis, joint pain, and joint effusion
– For acute rheumatic complaints
– For sore throat, tonsillitis
– For mastitis.

External Forms of Application
– As a quark compress or wrapped compress.

Contraindication milk protein allergy [8]

7.1.17 Marigold Flowers: *Calendulae Flos*

Plant Family Asteraceae

Species *calendula officinalis*

Origin Europe

Composition flavonoids, triterpene saponins, carotenoids, essential oil, coumarins, bitter compounds, polysaccharides

Brief Overview of Tradition as a Remedy Marigold flowers have been used as components in folk medicines since the Middle Ages. Taken internally against poisoning (worms), as a diaphoretic, diuretic, decongestant in digestive disorders, and liver disorders. Applied externally for tumors and inflammations, gynecological disorders, menstrual cramps, or to induce menstruation (Fig. 7.7).

Effects
– Wound-healing
– Anti-inflammatory
– Analgesic
– Antibacterial
– Stimulation of the lymphatic flow
– Skin caring.

Fig. 7.7 Marigold [1]

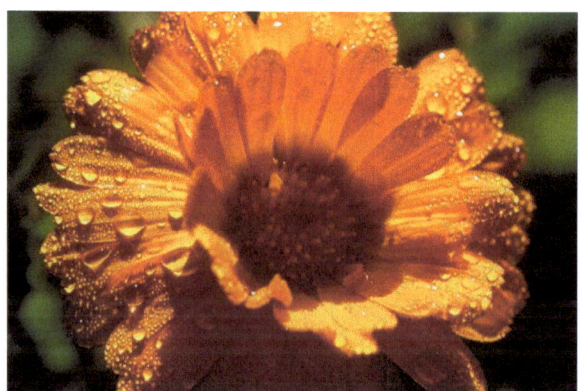

Range of Use
Internal
– For digestive problems.

External
– For skin inflammations, small superficial wounds and abrasions
– For poorly healing wounds, bruises, lacerations and defect wounds, and for first-degree decubitus ulcers
– For babies in case of soreness on the buttocks area and diaper rash
– In case of inflammatory changes of the oral and pharyngeal mucosa
– For burns or frostbite of the skin
– For nipple care for nursing mothers.

External Forms of Application
– As a tea infusion, e.g., for compresses or wound irrigation
– As a tincture (always use diluted)
– As oil for embrocation
– As ointment or cream, e.g., wound ointment (from Weleda).

Contraindication   allergy to the ingredients, allergy to cruciferous vegetables [2, 4]

7.1.18 Rose Petals: *Rosae Flos*

Plant Family   Rosaceae

Species   *rosa damascena, gallica, centifolia, alba*

Origin   Greater Persia/Iran

Composition   essential oil, tannins, lipids, wax, resin

Brief Overview of Tradition as a Remedy   The Greeks attributed the origins of the rose, the so-called "flower of love," to the Greek goddess Aphrodite. For over 5000 years, the plant has been used as a remedy, for example, as an infusion against diarrhea or as a mouthwash, and to gargle. In Persia, rose oil and rose water are taken for cramping stomach complaints and liver-bile colic.

Effects
– Astringent
– Antiseptic
– Anti-inflammatory.

Range of Use
External (only)
– For anxiety
– For chapped skin and cold sores on the lips
– For inflammations in the mouth and throat area
– For lack of strength and states of exhaustion
– For sleep disorders
– To support and enhance mood and in case of depression
– For nervous tension in the neck and back
– For heart problems caused by nervousness
– For mastitis.

External Forms of Application
– As a component of an oil (e.g., gold-rose-lavender oil, light earth), e.g., for a pentagram embrocation and others
– As a component of a cream (e.g., Aurum/Lavandula comp cream, Weleda,) e.g., for heart embrocation or compress.

Contraindication allergy to the ingredients [2, 4]

7.1.19 Rosemary Leaves: *Rosmarini Folium*

Plant Family Lamiaceae

Species *rosmarinus officinalis*

Origin Mediterranean area

Composition essential oil, tannins, rosmarinic acid

Brief Overview of Tradition as a Remedy In the first century, the Greek physician Dioscorides described rosemary as a medicinal plant that has warming powers, cures jaundice, and as an ingredient for ointments. It has been used since the sixteenth century in Europe to stimulate appetite and aid digestion, as well as an anti-flatulent and wound-healing agent (Fig. 7.8).

Effects
– Stimulates blood circulation
– Antispasmodic
– Antibacterial
– Antiviral
– Antioxidant.

Fig. 7.8 Rosemary [1]

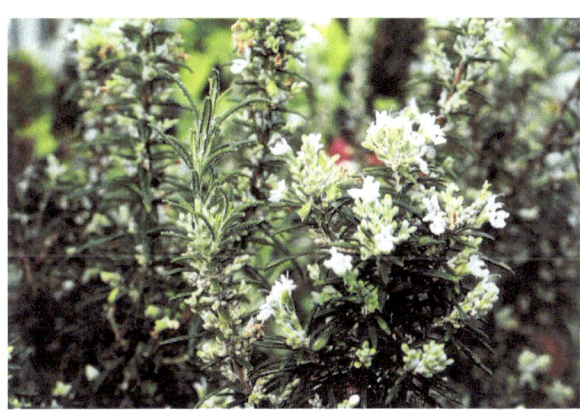

Range of Use
External (only)
- For mild cramp-like complaints in the gastrointestinal tract and dyspeptic complaints
- To improve the function of the liver and gallbladder
- For circulatory problems
- For states of exhaustion and fatigue
- For depression
- For restlessness and sleep disorders
- For cold legs and feet

External Forms of Application
- As an oily liniment for mild muscle and joint complaints
- As bath milk, e.g., for footbaths (e.g., Rosemary Activating Bath, Weleda), for difficulties in falling asleep and staying asleep (do not use directly before going to bed!)
- As rosemary socks with rosemary ointment 1% (see Chap. 6 Indications), e.g., for premature infants with mild bradycardia/apnea syndrome.

Contraindication allergy to the ingredients [2, 4]

Note The essential oil contains camphor and should always be diluted before use. Do not use during pregnancy, and in babies and toddlers up to 3 years (exception: Rosemary Socks, see Chap. 6).

7.1.20 Sea Buckthorn: *Hippophae Rhamnoides L.*

Plant Family Elaeagnaceae

Species *hippohae*

Part of the Plant Used Berries

Origin Eurasia, Central Europe

Composition vitamin B12, vitamin C, vitamin E, beta-carotene, fruit oil, tannins, flavonoids

Brief Overview of Tradition as a Remedy Sea buckthorn originally comes from the Himalayan Mountains in Nepal. Around 1400, the plant was mentioned in Europe for the first time. In the Middle Ages, monks and Hildegard von Bingen, the German Benedictine abbess known as St. Hildegard in the eleventh century, used sea buckthorn pulp as a remedy. In Eastern Europe, sea buckthorn has a long healing tradition. In World War II, sea buckthorn was taken to supply vitamin C (Fig. 7.9).

Effects
– Antibacterial
– Astringent
– Anti-inflammatory
– Analgesic
– Wound-healing.

Fig. 7.9 Sea Buckthorn [1]

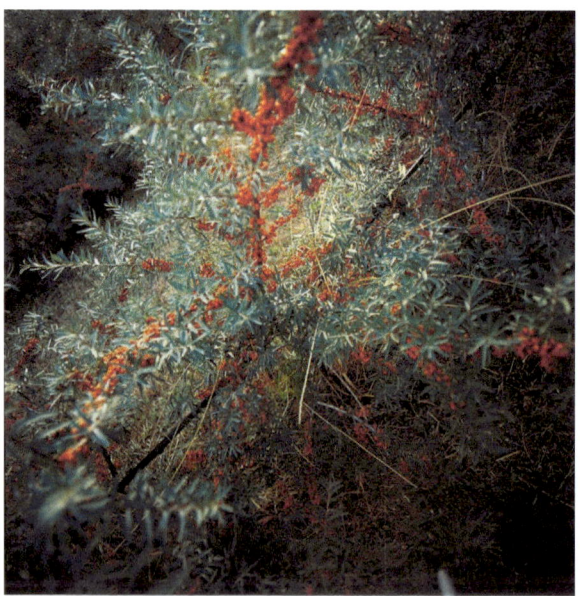

Range of Use
Internal
– For vitamin C deficiency
– For convalescence
– For colds.

External
– For 1st degree burns
– For oral care in case of aphthae and ulcers
– For skin and mucous membrane inflammations.

External Forms of Application
– As sea buckthorn pulp oil for oral care
– Dissolved in a carrier oil for skin care.

Contraindication allergy to the ingredients [3]

7.1.21 Yarrow: *Millefolii Herba*

Plant Family Asteraceae

Species *achillea millefolium*

Origin Europe

Composition essential oil, chamazulene, bitter substances, flavonoids, and tannins

Brief Overview of Tradition as a Remedy In ancient times, the Greek physician Dioscorides described yarrow as an agent for wound healing, anti-inflammatory, and hemostatic. In the Middle Ages, the Benedictine abbess Hildegard von Bingen used yarrow to heal wounds and for "three-day fever." From the seventeenth to the nineteenth centuries in Europe, the plant was used as a "cure-all" and for general invigoration. Traditionally, yarrow is used for cardiovascular diseases.

Effects
– Antibacterial
– Antispasmodic
– Digestive, cholagogue
– Astringent
– Anti-inflammatory
– Granulation-promoting
– Antioxidant.

Range of Use
Internal
- For loss of appetite
- For mild gastrointestinal cramps and flatulence.

External
- For constipation
- For loss of appetite, nausea, and vomiting
- For restlessness and anxiety
- For sleep disorders
- For states of exhaustion, listlessness, and depression
- For superficial wounds, skin and mucous membrane inflammations
- For soreness on the buttocks
- During and after chemotherapy
- For pneumonias.

External Forms of Application
- As a tea infusion for compresses, e.g., for chemotherapy, anxiety, liver diseases, states of exhaustion, sleep disorders, and as an additive in sitting baths for inflammations of the skin and mucous membrane in the buttock area
- Plant extracts and essential oil dissolved in a carrier oil (fatty vegetable oil) for embrocation (e.g., yarrow massage oil, lichterde oil), e.g., supportive for neonatal jaundice.

Contraindication Allergy to the ingredients [2, 4]

7.1.22 Mustard Seeds, Black: *Sinapis Nigrae Semen*

Plant Family Brassicaceae

Species *brassica nigra*

Origin Mediterranean area, Eastern Europe

Composition 30% fatty oil, pungent substances: mustard glycosides, sinigrin, flavonoids, phytin and mucilage

Brief Overview of Tradition as a Remedy Starting 3000 years ago, mustard found common use in China as a spice for adding flavor to food. In ancient times, mustard flour was used as a skin irritant for joint inflammation, rheumatic complaints, bronchitis, and pneumonia.

Effects
- Stimulating
- Stimulates blood circulation
- Activation of metabolic processes
- Antibacterial
- Anti-inflammatory
- Analgesic
- Wound-healing
- Expectorant.

Range of Use:
External (only)
- For bronchitis or pneumonia
- At the onset of flu with headache
- For cystitis
- For nerve pain
- For muscle tension
- For rheumatic complaints
- For migraines
- For chronic asthmatic complaints.

External Forms of Application
- As a mustard flour compress and wrapped compress, e.g., for bronchitis or pneumonia
- As a mustard flour foot bath, e.g., for oncoming flu, colds, and headaches.

Contraindication Hypersensitivity reactions, in case of open wounds and sensitive skin

Note Mustard flour has a strong skin irritating effect and can cause burns and blistering [2, 5].

7.1.23 Tea Tree oil: *Melaleuca Aetheroleum*

Plant Family Myrtaceae

Species *Melaleuca Alternifolia*

Origin Australia

Composition essential oil, terpinen-4-ol, 1.8-cineole, isoprenoids, cyclic monoterpenes, sesquiterpenes, alcohols

Brief Overview of Tradition as a Remedy Tea tree oil, native to the Australian Continent, has been used for centuries by the aboriginal people, for colds, sore throats, and for the treatment of wounds and insect bites. Since the eighteenth century, it has also been known in the Western world as a "cure-all."

Effects
– Antibacterial, antifungal, and antiviral
– Anti-inflammatory
– Antioxidant.

Range of Use
External (only)
– For cold sores
– For superficial wounds
– For inflammation of the oral mucosa.

External Forms of Application
– In shea butter, e.g., as lip care for dry lips, aphthae, or herpes labialis
– As mouth balm

Contraindication allergy to the ingredients, in allergic contact dermatitis, do not use on the eye [2, 3]

7.1.24 *Thyme* (Herb): *Thymi Herba*

Plant Family Lamiaceae

Species *thymus vulgaris*

Origin Mediterranean area, Southern Europe, Balkans, Caucasus, East Africa, India, Turkey, Israel, Morocco, North America

Composition essential oil: thymol, carvacrol, labiate tannins, flavonoids, triterpenes

Brief Overview of Tradition as a Remedy Thyme was used by the Sumerians more than 4000 years ago as a medicinal spice plant. Medical history shows tyme was used as an expectorant and for use in "wheezing and coughing." German abbess and healer Hildegard von Bingen recommended thyme for respiratory and gastrointestinal diseases. In European folk medicine, thyme is used as an antispasmodic stomachic, diuretic, flatulence, urinary disinfectant, and worm remedy (Fig. 7.10).

Fig. 7.10 Thyme [1]

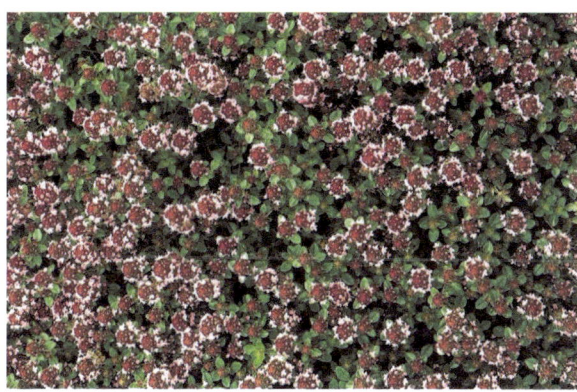

Effects
– Ejecting
– Expectorant
– Anti-inflammatory
– Antibacterial
– Antiviral
– Antifungal
– Dilates the bronchi
– Stimulates blood circulation.

Range of Use
Internal
– Expectorant for coughs caused by colds and inflammation of the mucous membranes of the upper respiratory tract
– For sore throat, persistent cough, and acute bronchitis.

External
– For the relief of cold symptoms
– For inflammation of the respiratory tract
– For inflammation of the oral mucosa and against bad breath
– For urinary tract infections and cystitis.

External Forms of Application
– As tea infusion for baths, e.g., sitz bath for urinary tract infections
– Dissolved in oil in a cold bath
– As a mouthwash preparation for inflammations of the oral mucosa
– As a tea infusion, e.g., for chest compresses for coughs
– As essential oil, e.g., for room diffusion in case of pseudo-croup

Contraindication allergy to the ingredients, in case of hypersensitivity reactions [2]

7.1.25 Wood Sorrel: *Oxalis Acetosella*

Plant Family Oxalidaceae

Species *oxalis acetosella*

Origin Central Europe and Eurasia

Composition potassium oxalate, oxalic acid, anthraquinone

Brief Overview of Tradition as a Remedy Since ancient times, wood sorrel has been used in many ways as a medicinal plant, including as a paste for ulcers, as an extract for heartburn, diarrhea, and indigestion, and as dried herb against poisoning, hemostasis, and scurvy (Fig. 7.11).

Range of Use
External (only)
– For abdominal embrocation in constipation, flatulence, and colic in infants
– For abdominal cramps
– For acute and chronic gastrointestinal diseases
– For vomiting
– For sleep disorders
– In case of fear, shock (mental) and trauma.

External Forms of Application:
– As a compress/wrapped compress with Oxalis ointment (e.g., from Weleda) or Oxalis essence (e.g., from Wala)

Contraindication allergy to the ingredients [3, 4]

Fig. 7.11 Wood sorrel [1]

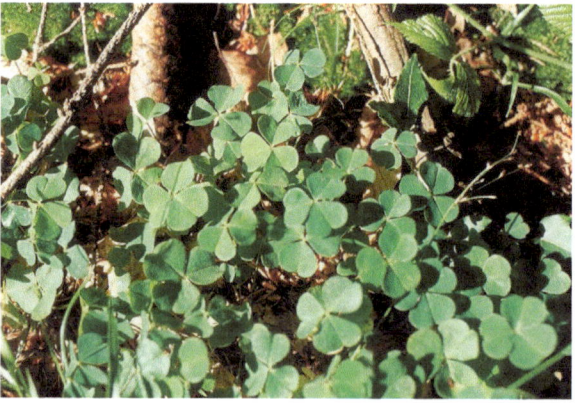

7.1.26 Wild Pansy with Flowers: *Violae herba cum flore*

Plant Family Violaceae

Species *Viola tricolor*

Origin Europe, Asia

Composition flavonoids: violanthin, salicylates; mucilages, tannins, essential oil, coumarins, carotenoids, vitamin C.

Brief Overview of Tradition as a Remedy Used as an external application for itching, rashes and head colds in children since the sixteenth century in Europe. Also used for catarrh of the respiratory tract, whooping cough, sore throat, and feverish colds as a "blood purifier". In traditional medicine, pansy is used as a diuretic, diaphoretic, and laxative, as well as for rheumatism, gout, and arteriosclerosis.

Effects
– Anti-inflammatory
– Analgesic
– Antibacterial.

Range of Use
External (only)
– For itching with eczema, neurodermatitis, and allergy
  For cradle cap and diaper dermatitis.

External Forms of Application
– As a tea infusion, e.g., for itch-reducing whole-body washing
– As a bath additive, e.g., for neurodermatitis.

Contraindication allergy to the ingredients [3, 6]

7.1.27 Cistus Leaves: *Cistus Incanus*

Plant Family Cistaceae

Species *cistus incanus*

Origin Mediterranean area

Composition monoterpenes 40–50% monoterpenols 5–15%, esters 5–15%, sesquiterpenes 5–10%, sesquiterpenols 5%, monoterpene ketones 4–7%, monoterpene aldehydes 3–5%, eugenol up to 1.5%

Brief Overview of Tradition as a Remedy Endemic to the Mediterranean, cistus has been used as a medicinal plant for over 2000 years. The leaves and stems are used for infections and diarrhea, as well as skin diseases.

Effects
– Anti-inflammatory
– Antibacterial
– Antiviral
– Cell regenerating, wound healing, and blood circulation enhancing
– Decongesting, promoting lymph flow.

Range of Use
Internal
– For neurodermatitis and itching
– For flu-like infections and colds.

External
– For (cut) wounds
– For hematomas
– For lymphatic congestion.

External Forms of Application
– As essential oil dissolved in carrier oil, e.g., for hematomas
– As a tea infusion for washes for atopic dermatitis.

Contraindication allergy to the ingredients and hypersensitivity [3, 6]

7.1.28 Lemon Peel: *Citri Pericarpium*

Plant Family Rutaceae

Species *citrus limon*

Origin Mediterranean area, Africa, Caribbean Islands

Composition essential oil: limonene, flavonoids, carotenoids, and citric acid

Brief Overview of Tradition as a Remedy Lemon was cultivated in China from 500 BC onward. In the thirteenth century, it reached Europe with the crusaders. In the seventeenth century, the Scottish ship's doctor James Lind used citric acid on his sailors against scurvy (Fig. 7.12).

Fig. 7.12 Lemon
(fruit) [1]

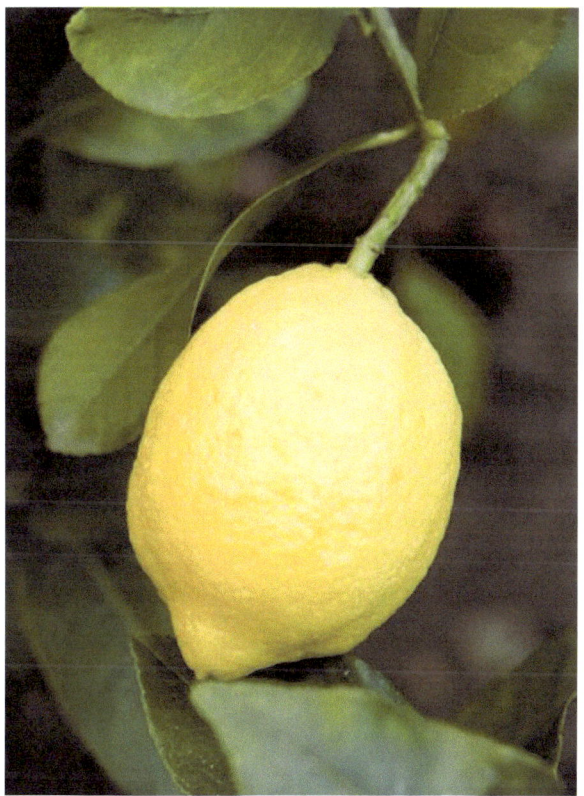

Effects
– Antioxidant
– Astringent
– Decongestant
– Expectorant
– Antipyretic
– Anti-inflammatory
– Analgesic
– Diuretic
– Invigorating and refreshing.

Range of Use
Internal

– To support the digestive function
– For flu-like infections
– For allergic diseases.

194

C. Oberle

External
- For fever
- To improve the malaise
- For nausea
- For loss of appetite
- For sore throat
- For exhaustion
- For flu-like infections
- For pneumonias
- For bronchitis
- For heart problems.

External Forms of Application
- Essential oil of lemon used as a water additive for a whole body wash, for example, in case of fever
- As a throat compress with lemon slices, e.g., for beginning sore throats, tonsillitis, pharyngitis, laryngitis, and flu-like infections
- Lemon slices for a foot compress, e.g., for fever
- As a chest compress for bronchitis
- As footbath.

Contraindication allergy to the ingredients, hypersensitive reactions [2, 6]

7.1.29 Onion: *Allii Cepae Bulbus*

Plant Family Alliaceae

Species *allium cepa*

Origin Central Asia

Composition sulfur-containing compounds, alliin, peptides and flavonoids

Brief Overview of Tradition as a Remedy The onion is an ancient, widespread cultivated plant, found in the household of both the Egyptians and the Romans since ancient times. As a medicinal plant, it is used for infectious diseases, insect bites, cough, cold, or earache.

Effects
- Antibacterial
- Anti-inflammatory
- Analgesic.

Range of Use
Internal

– For loss of appetite
– For sore throat
– For cough
– For allergies.

External

– For otitis media
– For bee and wasp stings
– For cough.

External Forms of Application
(Chopped)
– As onion sachets/compresses for earache and for middle ear infection
– As a chest compress for incipient cough
– As a compress for bee and wasp stings.

Contraindication allergy to the ingredients, hypersensitive reactions [5, 6]

7.2   Ready-to-Use Preparations

The following describes over-the-counter preparations that we recommend for external applications. The preparations can be obtained from pharmacies or from the manufacturer itself (see supply sources).

7.2.1   Aconite Pain Oil (Wala)

Active Substances
– Potentiated monkshood
– Lavender oil
– Real camphor.

Form of Application:
– As a wrapped compress/compress/embrocation in a body area with pain

Contraindication Do not use in children under 6 years or in cases of hypersensitivity to the ingredients and camphor, soy, peanut.

7.2.2   Aloe Vera Oil, Organic

Active Substances
– Aloe vera extract

Form of Application   see Aloe Vera

Contraindication   hypersensitivity to the ingredients

7.2.3   Arnica Essence (Wala; Weleda)

Active Substances
– Wala: Arnica montana e floribus LA 20%
– Weleda: Arnica, Planta tota mother tincture

Form of Application   see arnica flowers

Contraindication   Do not use in case of hypersensitivity to the ingredients of the preparation such as chamomile flowers, calendula, and yarrow or in case of damaged skin.

Note   Do not use pure, always dilute with water

7.2.4   Arnica Massage Oil (Weleda)

Active Substances
– Arnica montana extract

Form of Application   see arnica flowers

Contraindication   hypersensitivity to the ingredients

7.2.5   Aurum/Lavandula Comp. Cream (Weleda)

Active substances
– Aurum metallicum praeparatum D4
– Lavender oil
– Rose petal extract.

Uses
– For heart complaints, palpitations, cardiac anxiety, and cardiac arrhythmias
– For circulatory problems
– In palliative care.

Form of Application
- As an embrocation (e.g., heart or pentagram embrocation) or as a heart ointment compress

Contraindication Hypersensitivity to the ingredients according to the technical information.

7.2.6 Calendula Wound Ointment (Weleda)

Active Substances
- Calendula officinalis 2a mother tincture

Form of Application see Marigold Flowers

Contraindication Hypersensitivity to the ingredients as listed in the instructions for use/content information (including lanolin and lanolin alcohols).

7.2.7 Eucalyptus, Oleum Aethereum 10% (Wala)

Active Substances
- Eucalyptus oil 10%

Form of Application see eucalyptus leaves

Contraindication Do not use in case of hypersensitivity to the ingredients listed in the instructions for use/content information.

7.2.8 Fennel-Cumin Oil for Children (Bahnhof-Apotheke)

Active Substances
- Anise, fennel, coriander, and cumin
- Almond and evening primrose oil

Application
- For digestive disorders of the gastrointestinal tract, three-month colic in babies, abdominal pain, and constipation

Application Form
- For abdominal rubbing or as an oil application, e.g., for abdominal cramps, flatulence, and constipation

Contraindication hypersensitivity to the ingredients

7.2.9   Gold Rose Lavender Massage Oil (Uriel)

Active Substances
– Gold leaf
– Rose petal extract, rose oil
– Lavender oil

Application
– For anxiety and restlessness
– For problems with falling and staying asleep
– For exhaustion, listlessness and depression
– For worry and circles of thought
– For panic attacks
– For stress
– In palliative situations.

Form of Application: Oily Liniment
– As a rub for the back, calves, hands, and feet, e.g., for anxiety and restlessness, sleep problems, and exhaustion
– As a pentagram rub in terminal care.

Contraindication Hypersensitivity to the ingredients according to the ingredient list.

7.2.10 Hypericum ex Herba 5% (Wala)

Active Substances
– St. John's Wort oil 5%

Form of Application see St. John's Wort

Contraindication children under 6 years; hypersensitivity to the ingredients (including peanut) listed in the instructions for use/content information

7.2.11 Immortelle Water, hydrolate bio

Active Substances
– Immortelle hydrolate

Form of Application see Immortelle

Contraindication Hypersensitivity to the ingredients according to the ingredient list.

7.2.12 Copper Ointment Red (Wala)

Active Substances
– Copper oxide

Uses
– For cold conditions of hands and feet

Form of Application
– As an embrocation

Contraindication Hypersensitivity to the ingredients according to the instructions for use.

7.2.13 Lavender Relaxing Care Oil (Weleda)

Active Substances:
– Lavender oil

Form of Application see Lavender Flowers

Contraindication Hypersensitivity to the ingredients according to the ingredient list.

7.2.14 Lavender Relaxing Bath (Weleda)

Active Substances
– Lavender oil

Form of Application see Lavender Flowers

Contraindication Hypersensitivity to the ingredients according to the ingredient list.

7.2.15 Lavender Oil 10% (Weleda)

Active Substances
– Lavender oil

Application form see Lavender Flowers

Contraindication Hypersensitivity to the ingredients according to the ingredients list

7.2.16 Mallow Oil (Wala)

Active Substances
– Mallow
– Black elderberry
– Sloe flowers
– St. John's Wort
– Lime blossoms
– Geranium essential oil.

Application form see Mallow Flowers

Contraindication Hypersensitivity to the ingredients (including peanut, soy) according to the list of ingredients.

7.2.17 Medihoney

Active Substances
– Medicinal Manuka honey (CE certified, medical device class IIb)

Effect
– Antibacterial and antifungal
– Disinfecting
– Anti-inflammatory
– Wound-healing
– Antioxidant
– Odor eliminating.

Application
External
– As a medicinal honey and wound gel.
– For infected wounds, acute or chronic wounds
– For deep wounds and decubitus grade III
– For wounds with multiple resistant germs (MRSA)
– For burns
– For skin diseases such as psoriasis
– For navel care in newborns.

Form of Application
– The wound gel is mainly used for superficial wounds, such as abrasions or for wound care at catheter exit sites
– For wound cleansing and wound care.

Contraindication in case of hypersensitivity to bee products and to the listed ingredients

7.2.18 Melissa oil (Wala)

Active Substances
- Melissa oil
- Caraway oil
- Bitter fennel oil
- Marjoram oil.

Uses
- For anxiety, restlessness, irritability, and tension
- For states of exhaustion
- For abdominal cramps and flatulence.

Form of Application
- As an embrocation or oil compress

Contraindication in case of hypersensitivity to the ingredients (including peanut oil and soy) according to the list of ingredients

7.2.19 Oxalis Essence (Wala)

Active Substances
- Oxalis acetosella e planta tota LA 20%

Form of Application see Wood Sorrel

Contraindication Hypersensitivity to the ingredients according to the list of ingredients

7.2.20 Oxalis Folium 10% Ointment (Weleda)

Active Substances
- Oxalis acetosella, folium mother tincture

Form of Application see Wood Sorrel

Contraindication Hypersensitivity to the ingredients (including wool wax and wool wax alcohols) according to the list of ingredients

7.2.21 Propolis Tincture 20%

Active Substances
– Propolis

Form of Application see Propolis

Contraindication allergy to bee products and ingredients.

7.2.22 Rosemary Activating Bath (Weleda)

Active substances
– Rosemary oil
– Limonene
– Linalool

Form of Application see Rosemary Leaves

Contraindication hypersensitivity reaction and to the ingredients

7.2.23 Sea Buckthorn Organic 100% Pulp Oil

Active Substances
– Sea buckthorn pulp oil

Form of Application see Sea Buckthorn

Contraindication hypersensitivity reaction to the ingredients of the oil

7.2.24 Yarrow Massage Oil

Active Substances
– Extract from yarrow flowers
– Yarrow essential oil

Form of Application see yarrow herb

Contraindication hypersensitivity reaction to the ingredients.

7.2.25 Shea Butter Raw & Organic

Active Substances
– Butyrospermum Parkii Butter

Uses
– As a base for lip balm or nose ointment

Contraindication hypersensitivity reaction to the ingredients of shea butter

7.2.26 Solum Oil (Wala):

Active Substances:
– Raised bog peat
– Horse chestnut
– Field horsetail
– Lavender oil.

Uses
– For weather sensitivity
– For anxiety and restlessness
– For pain, chronic pain, and nerve pain
– For sleep problems
– Supportive in rheumatic diseases
– Supportive for tumor and metastasis pain.

Form of Application
– As an embrocation for the back, calves, hands and feet, e.g., for pain, anxiety, and restlessness

Contraindication inflammations and injuries of the skin; hypersensitivity to the ingredients (including lanolin and lanolin alcohols) according to the list of ingredients

7.3   Base Oils

Pure vegetable oils such as olive oil, almond oil, or sunflower oil are used as base oils. They can be used pure or mixed as a carrier oil with essential oils or other components for the respective indication.

7.4   Supply Sources

The products listed are considered to be of high quality and are recommended for medical use based on their use in scientific studies.

https://www.primaveralife.com/international

https://www.walaarzneimittel.de/de/ueber-wala/wala-international.html

https://www.weleda.com/international

https://shop.bahnhof-apotheke.de/product/fenchel-kuemmel-oel-fuer-kinder-50ml.320

https://shopuriel.com/

https://truebotanica.com

References

1. 2021 Photographs © Weleda AG
2. Wichtl (2015) Teedrogen und Phytopharmaka: Ein Handbuch für die Praxis. [Tea drugs and phytopharmaceuticals: a handbook for practice] (Wissenschaftliche Verlagsgesellschaft), Stuttgart
3. Scripts of the additional training: Qualification naturopathic care for children by Gisela Blaser
4. Sommer M (2018) Heilpflanzen: Ihr Wesen - ihre Wirkung - ihre Anwendung [Medicinal plants: their essence - their effect - their application] (Aethera) 3rd ed
5. Heine R (2015) Anthroposophische Pflegepraxis: Grundlagen und Anregungen für alltägliches Handeln: Grundlagen und Anregungen für alltägliches Handeln [Anthroposophical nursing practice: fundamentals and suggestions for everyday action] (Salumed) 3rd ed
6. Huber M (2014) Complementary medicine, 1st ed
7. https://www.pflege-vademecum.de/quark.php
8. Meadow G (1996) Neurodermatitis treatment with Cystus tea herb. Naturopathic Pract Nat Med 49:1069–1071